Bob Martel has done it again with another fabulous book! The U.S. population has gone from an average of 8.5 hours of sleep per night in 1950 to an abysmal 6.5 hours in 2020 with catastrophic effects to our health, safety, productivity and longevity. Bob gives us a roadmap with detailed instructions on how to easily get the sleep we need for optimum health. It is the best book I have ever read on this subject and I have read them all!

    —John Asher, CEO of Asher Strategies and The Asher Longevity Institute, and Author of *Close Deals Faster*, *The Neuroscience of Selling*, and *The Future of Sales*

This book is AMAZING! As a leading expert in professional hypnosis, I thought I knew a lot about sleep. But Bob Martel is literally the Rip Van Winkle in teacher form, here to guide you into gentle nights of blissful sleep. I learned some great things about how to sleep using the advice in this book, and you will too! No wonder they call Bob the sleep whisperer!

    —Dr. Richard Nongard, Professional Hypnotist, Author & President of the International Certification Board of Clinical Hypnotists

Bob Martel has penned another book that gives you simple, practical, and real answers to life's challenges. This time, it's all about sleep. Sleep is something you and I both need more of and Bob shows you how to do it without needing to spend money on anything.

    —Dr. Kevin Hogan, Author of *The New Hypnotherapy Handbook*, and *The Psychology of Persuasion*

Sleep is the healthiest thing we can do for ourselves. Robert (Bob) Martel is a specialist at taking you into that simply wonderful state. Allow him to guide you back to sleep in an easy method that worked for me and many others. I wish I had this book years ago.

    —Richard Green, Captain, Kalamazoo Sheriff Dept. (Retired), Board Certified Hypnotherapist

Inspired by his unique life experiences Bob Martel brings to light common-sense approaches to naturally fall and stay asleep without the aid of medication or devices, just by using the ability within that we all possess. His often-witty personal stories, trials and tribulations with time distortion in the military as a submariner and flying around the world in his corporate life help us to understand that sleep is attainable with the correct mindset and methods. I've been using Bob's techniques for many years and I have had much better quality of sleep, and am able to fall asleep quickly and effortlessly every night. For anyone who struggles with sleep nightly or occasionally, this book is a game-changer!

> —Lori Braverman, Professional Hypnotist, ABO-Certified Optician

Robert Martel is a master hypnotist and storyteller who will take you on a journey into sleep through the wealth of wisdom he shares in *I Am Sleeping Now*. In this book you will examine what has been keeping you awake, and find techniques you need to create your own personal method of easily falling asleep. He invites you through his words to use your imagination in setting positive intentions to accomplish your sleeping goals which could lead to some incredible positive changes in many aspects of your life. Enjoy the journey, and sleep well.

> —Michael Hathaway, Author of *The Everything Lucid Dreaming Book*, *The Everything Hypnosis Book*, and *It's Time to Simplify Your Soul's Code*

In today's fast-paced and action-packed world, who knew that those who sleep a third of their life away were actually the lucky ones. This book is what dreams are made of and is a must-have for anyone looking to live life with energy. I never realized how much you had to know to be good at doing nothing, but Bob Martel has put together the exact strategy to do just that and in turn make the waking hours of your day amazing.

> —Rich Guzzi, Professional Hypnotist, Coach, Entrepreneur, and Author of the book *Performing Hypnosis: How to Captivate an Audience of One or a Thousand and Everything in Between*

A must-read book! If you or anyone you know is struggling getting a restful sleep this book is the answer. Bob Martel's clear, concise, easy to read and follow book *I Am Sleeping Now* gives you the emotional, physical, and practical tools to achieve a peaceful and restful sleep. Enjoy it!

—Debbie Papadakis, Registered Psychotherapist, Clinical Hypnotherapist, Relationship Coach, Sleep Deprivation Specialist, NLP/Time-Line Therapy Trainer, Author of the book *The Relationship Code*

Better performance in work and life comes down to a few fundamental practices. But the key practice that provides out-sized results when it comes to attitude, effectiveness, and results is sleep. Getting seven hours of good sleep, and you are the Dali Lama. Five hours of bad sleep and you are something close to Joseph Stalin. Read *I Am Sleeping Now* and get the rest you deserve. Remember, in the working world, Monday starts on Sunday, and a good night's sleep sets you up for success!

—Anthony Iannarino, Internationally Recognized Corporate Sales Coach, Speaker and Trainer, Author of *Eat Their Lunch: Winning Customers Away from Your Competition*, and *The Only Sales Guide You'll Ever Need*

Imagine reading a book that puts you to sleep! It is not too appealing unless you have trouble sleeping. We all know that sleep is central to our physical health, emotional well-being, and achievement. Bob offers practical, easily implemental strategies for sleep that will enhance your waking hours. His sleep strategies work for all ages!

—Gerry Dougherty, President, Boston Independence Group, Inc., Author of *Uncomplicated Money*

For those of us who struggle with getting restful sleep, Bob Martel's book is a gift. He generously shares his wisdom and precise instructions on how to shift from sleeplessness and insomnia to drug-free sleep. For skeptics, he even offers a Seven-Day Sleep Improvement Challenge to test the strategies he outlines in his *I Am Sleeping Now* book.

—Susan Bellows, Human Resource Consultant

Realizing your full potential in business and in life requires that you develop excellent sleep skills, attitudes and habits. This book teaches you how to condition your mind and body to easily enjoy better sleep. Watch your business soar with the masterful techniques Bob shares in this book... even while you're asleep!

—Jason Linett, Best-Selling Author of *Work Smart Business*, Host of the *Hypnotic Language Hacks*™ Podcast

The power of these two simple words "I Am," have proven themselves time and time again to be life-changing. We are and attract into our lives what we choose to think, say and believe about ourselves, and our perceived reality. In this amazing and well laid out book, you will learn exactly how to control your mind and body to achieve a deep and fulfilling level of sleep. You will soon learn that the power of "I Am" can easily be incorporated into all aspects of one's life, and this book is the perfect place to start.

—R. J. Banks, Author of *The Power of I AM and the Law of Attraction*

Bob Martel has written an easy-to-read, engaging, and surprisingly effective book. I describe the book as "surprising," because if you just skipped over it, you might come to the conclusion that the system contained within is simplistic and naive. You could not be more wrong! As you work through the book, following the various exercises, progressing as the book does, you may come to the same unavoidable conclusion I did — this stuff really works.

—Graham Old, Professional Hypnotist, Author of *Let It Be*

Bob has done it again! This follow-up to *The Magic of Aesop* is an easy read filled with ways to get you to sleep rather than the usual explanations or reasons you can't sleep and to top it off the tools he provides are easy to learn and incorporate into your daily routines. This will be a recommended read for all future clients who are dealing with sleep issues. Very well done, Bob.

—Anthony Gitch, CONTROL Practitioner | Remedial Hypnotist

Getting a good night's sleep on a regular basis is critical for well-being. In this book, *I Am Sleeping Now*, by Bob Martel, you will see that Bob has dialed into the solution for getting a full night of restorative sleep through the use of self-hypnosis. Bob's experience as an author and a professional hypnotist blend together to deliver the optimal solution for the very unpleasant experience of sleep deprivation. If you are looking for a natural effective way to improve your sleep experience you have come to the right place.

 —Debbie Taylor, Intuitive Life Coach & Author

Bob Martel's book *I Am Sleeping Now* reminds us of some really important factors-to slow down, unplug and settle into rituals that not only improve our sleep, but our focus and functioning overall. In today's world of technology, devices, and chaos, relaxation and sleep are even more imperative. *I Am Sleeping Now* gives us all of the tools and exercises needed to make changes and/or improvements for sleep, overall wellness and a positive outlook for tomorrow. Sound and quality sleep are a necessity to everyone. As a person with a sleep disorder, not only did Bob Martel's book remind us of the importance of relaxation and sleep, but it gave us the tools and techniques to improve and lead us into healthier daily rituals. His words on the significance of self-hypnosis and relaxation so we can start out each new day refreshed and ready for what awaits us were beyond significant. As E. Joseph Cossman (entrepreneur and author) said, "The best bridge between despair and hope is a good night's sleep." I think you'll enjoy reading this life-changing book.

 —Cindy McAnaney, LSW, MHRT-C

A major percentage of the clients in my clinical hypnotherapy practice have some degree of regular difficulty with sleep and often enough, a sleep deficit plays a significant role in creating the problems they wish to address. In *I Am Sleeping Now*, Martel presents easy, practical steps for self-help with sleep issues. I'd recommend this book to anyone even before considering over-the-counter or prescription sleep aids. The best better sleep self-help book. I'll certainly recommend it to my clients.

 —Joseph A. Onesta, Professional Hypnotist and Author of
 The Hypnofasting Program Guide

The twelve chapters and the seven steps to a good night's sleep outlined in this book provide the reader with the emotional intelligence and mindset for all readers to achieve the good night's sleep you deserve. The writer teaches you how to invite sleep in by building good foundations of sleep hygiene and a mindset of "I can" so you take control, put yourself in charge to achieve a wonderful hypnotic sleep. Even jet lag will become a thing of the past when you learn the magic formula within.

—Beryl Comar MA, MEd, MNLP, Emotional Intelligence Development Specialist, Author of the book *HypnoDontics*

In reading *I Am Sleeping Now*, I felt as if Bob were sitting there reading it to me. Through anecdote, personal experience, and a bit of background science, he creates a path to sleeping well, leading us in a way that we "already know how." By emphasizing practice of awareness instead of trying harder, personal presence instead of external intervention, and learning to keep separate things separate, he "walks the talk" of his clear, simple introduction: start where you are; accept without judgment what is true for you today.

—Bradford Glass, Life Coach, and Author of *Living Authentically*, and *A Field Guide to Life*

I have long admired my cousin Bob for his heart. From his service as a submariner in the U.S. Navy to his practice as a professional hypnotist he has dedicated his life to helping and protecting people. He hits a major league homerun with this book on sleep because he gives people the best gift of all: hope. He teaches the reader how to use the mind to rest the mind… and the body and spirit. From that rest comes renewal, strength, and purpose. The practical guidance and coaching he gives here will change your life. We all need more sleep, and Bob's natural, drug-free method works!

—Tom Martel, Playwright, Songwriter, Model Citizen

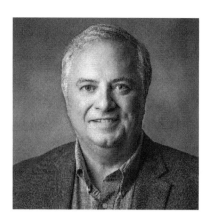

Meet the Author

Robert Martel is a Professional Clinical Hypnotist in private practice at Positive Results Hypnosis, in Holden, MA, which he founded in 2008. Bob is also a performance and confidence coach to business professionals and athletes who want to take their game, in business or in life, to the next level. He is a certified NLP practitioner and Life Coach through the ICBCH. Bob also founded a direct marketing consulting group in 1992 where he specialized in direct marketing and copywriting, serving clients in numerous industries using hypnotic influence and persuasion techniques to help clients to profitably grow their business. He provides clinical hypnosis services at his office and over the internet, serving clients worldwide.

As America's Leading Hypnotic Sleep Coach, Bob has worked with thousands of people to help them sleep better, enabling them to live a happier, more abundant and joyful life by using the power of their mind to connect with their God-given talents and gifts.

He is a graduate of Northeastern University, and a veteran of the U.S. Navy's Submarine Service. He is certified by the ICBCH as an NLP practitioner and Life Coach, and is an ICBCH and NGH-certified hypnosis instructor. He is also board-certified by the National Guild of Hypnotists. Bob is a commercial hot air balloon pilot, and resides in Central Massachusetts.

Do you want Bob to speak at your next event, provide private coaching, or to conduct a customized program for your company, or your team? Call (508)481-8383, visit www.positiveresultshypnosis, or email him at Bob@bobmartel.com, or visit his LinkedIn profile at LinkedIn.com/in/robertmartel

Additional Books by the Author

How to Create All of the Business You Can Handle: Smart Strategies for the Small Business Owner

"This book is really well suited for the small business owner who is trying to pull it all together and make it happen for his business, yet has few resources at his command."

 —Peter Hussey, CEO, Corestreet Ltd.

"No wonder they call Bob Martel the Velvet Sledge Hammer. In his soft style, he hits you over the head with powerful marketing strategies that apply to virtually any industry. Whether your interest is in the best way to take market share or how to make sure marketing improvements last, Bob spells it out."

 —Bill Evans, President, WorkSense Consulting Group

The Magic of Aesop: How to Use the Wisdom of Aesop's Fables to Spark Your Transformational Change

"This is the most significant and exciting book for hypnotherapists that I have read in a long time. I'm always looking for new ways of creating metaphors. I love how you teach the reader in your scripts. I've stared at my copy of Aesop's Fables many times and known that it's packed full of gems. This book is filled with powerful storytelling techniques which makes it useful as a continuing reference."

 —Roger Moore, Institute of Hypnotherapy

"This book is a must-have as it allows and teaches you through story telling how the client slowly but surely reassess and creates new choices on their own with your guidance. *The Magic of Aesop* is a wonderful resource book for helping many, many people to become the best version of themselves."

 —Patricia MacIsaac, DNGH, CMI, BCH, Owner of South Shore Hypnosis Center, Hingham, MA

I AM Sleeping NOW

HOW TO FALL ASLEEP, STAY ASLEEP AND WAKE UP REFRESHED

By
Robert Martel

A Seven Day Program that Puts You
on a Path to Enjoying Better Sleep

www.iamsleepingnow.com

I Am Sleeping Now:
How to Fall Asleep, Stay Asleep and Wake Up Refreshed

A Seven Day Program that Puts You on a Path to Enjoying Better Sleep

ISBN: 978-1-7354770-2-2

First printing July 2021

Positive Results Hypnosis
www.positiveresultshypnosis.com
www.iamsleepingnow.com

Robert Martel is available to speak at your business or conference event on a variety of topics, including sleep! Call him at (508) 481-8383 or inquire to bob@bobmartel.com for booking information or for corporate programs, or visit www.iamsleepingnow.com.

Note: All names of clients used in this book have been changed to protect client privacy.

Disclaimer: This book is not about the science of sleep, nor is it a book about *why* we sleep. This is a book that teaches you, the reader, how to easily fall asleep using the power of their own mind. This book is not intended to provide medical advice of any kind, nor does it provide any medical or alternative health recommendations regarding medication, nutrition, or supplements. Should the reader be seeking such advice, the author recommends consulting the appropriate medical and/or alternative health experts and resources. Further, this book does not provide any recommendations, assessments, or science pertaining to the study of sleep, sleep apnea, or a diagnosis of insomnia. A medical evaluation of insomnia may be appropriate, and this book does not attempt to diagnose or treat insomnia. The reader should seek professional medical attention for any of these symptoms or concerns.

Additionally, please know that I am not a sleep doctor, nor do I have any interest in selling mattresses, supplements, sleep monitoring technology or the like. This is not a book that offers any medical or pharmacological solutions. I am a professional hypnotist and hypnotists know how to help people enter that realm called sleep by conditioning the mind to sleep when sleep is what's next!

This book is dedicated to Hypnos, the god of sleep, and to all who have struggled throughout humanity to master the art of sleeping well!

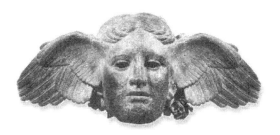

"Divine Hypnos, god who knows no pain,
Hypnos, stranger to anguish,
come in favor to us, come happy,
and giving happiness, great King!
Keep before his eyes such light as is spread before them now.
Come to him, I pray you, come with power to heal!"
—Sophocles, *Philoctetes* (409 B.C.)

"O, Hypnos,
divine repose of all things!
Gentlest of the deities!
Peace to the troubled mind,
from which you drive the cares of life.
Restorer of men's strength
when wearied with the toils of day."
—Ovid, *Metamorphoses*, Book XI (8 A.D.)

FOREWORD
By Michael R. Hathaway

At some point, nearly everyone has had an issue with getting enough sleep. It can be a nagging problem that affects your ability to live a fully productive life. As you delve into Robert Martel's masterful new book *I Am Sleeping Now*, you will be embarking on a journey to find out what has been causing your sleep issues and obtain tools for changing them. Robert Martel is a master of incorporating both neurolinguistics and storytelling into helping each reader of this easy-to-comprehend work understand their own lack of sleep story and how to rewrite it into one with a positive outcome. He does this by sharing his own stories, including learning to sleep in a submarine. His goals throughout this book are to encourage you to write your own "I Am Sleeping Now" story.

Let me share a little bit of how neurolinguistic programming literally changed my life. Following an accident in 1989, I found that it was hard for me to continue my career as a teacher. I had been actively using self-hypnosis for many years by that time, so I decided to prepare for a change in work and enrolled in a doctorate of clinical hypnosis program. The studies included an in-depth study of NLP. It was then that I learned to understand myself and how my mind worked, and it changed my life. There is a strong possibility that Robert Martel will help you do the same for your life.

So what is NLP? Simply, it is changing the language in your brain to create a new way of examining old non-productive thought patterns. Through story telling Robert helps you look at your life in terms of thinking and action patterns that let you discover things about yourself. As for myself, I had always felt that I did not know what people thought I knew. As a musician I could never play by ear and through NLP discovered I didn't recall sounds in my mind; I also found out I was non-visual and lacked the ability to reproduce the memory of taste, smell, or external touch. Now that I understand why I don't do what most others do, I use what comes easily to me instead. Robert will help you understand yourself. So how does this apply to sleep? There are many reasons people have trouble sleeping. It might be stress that you create yourself or that others create for you. It could be caused by one of your over-stimulated senses, interrupting what had been a good night's sleep. It could be related to your eating habits or a physical condition, such as pain, that gets in the way of relaxing enough to sleep. It may be your creative mind keeping you awake. It may be your dreams or nightmares. Robert deals with all of these concerns and so much more in *I Am Sleeping Now*.

In conclusion, I believe that this wonderful masterpiece could possibly change your life in many different ways. As you read his words, feel free to let your mind drift to your next thought. That is what Robert will help bring out of your subconscious mind. His words will go with you. Sleep well.

Michael R. Hathaway
Doctor of Clinical Hypnotherapy Madison, NH

PREFACE
Why Read This Book

Everyone deserves a good night's sleep, including you! That's the big reason for reading this book, to help you sleep well again, but let me say a bit more because this is a unique no-nonsense book about how to fall and stay asleep, and it's written for you!

You'll gain that edge in life that you're looking for, that *je ne sais quoi*, as the French say, that "I don't know what" — meaning that appealing thing, that certain something, that is difficult to describe and yet most pleasant and appreciated. You'll feel more alive again, with more energy to enjoy each day!

This book is all about a nonpharmacological approach to improving your sleep using your mind. Specifically, about how to fall asleep, go back to sleep, and wake up refreshed using self-hypnosis.

You are going to learn how to teach yourself how to sleep well again. Restful sleep will become again for you what it once was; your gateway to that new you, which is your old you, as you move your life forward one day at a time.

Know, as you begin your journey here in this book, that you should embrace any changes in small incremental steps as you invite sleep back into your life. Ease into the unique changes, the tiny shifts in your habitual rituals that will bring about the onset of sleep. You are here because change is necessary. Own it. Face it. Play with it. Learn from it. And enjoy that new you that emerges in this process.

If you are suffering from chronic sleep deficiency, this book will help you develop your personal action plan to make the changes you desire. And, hopefully, it will open your eyes to the dangers of long-term use of sleep medications as well, as you and your prescribing doctor have a conversation about medications and your sleep study results if chronic insomnia is suspected.

Every performance-improvement guru, business leader, and caregiver know that sleep is your secret weapon. Sleep is your performance X-factor — the invisible differentiator — and the elixir of life, or one of them anyway! It is as important as any physical and mental conditioning, nutrition, or skills development. In fact, sleeping well is a conditioned response to your intention (and from signals from the body), driven by your *intentions.* More on this later.

Let me ask forgiveness in advance if I mention this point a few times throughout this book: Sleep is the new 'exercise' and it is big business, as you probably already know. In fact, it is estimated to be a $30B market. Sleep technologists and venture capitalists are inventing new tools to measure our sleep, pseudo-doctors are hawking supplements and concoctions, and pharmaceutical companies are always dreaming up new pills. And, trust me, they are all staying up all night to compete for your money. *Caveat emptor.* Let the buyer beware.

There Is Only ONE Sleep Device You Need for Success – And It's Found Between Your Ears!

If you don't believe this quite yet, keep reading with an open mind. You do not need sleeping pills. The pills, or the myriad expensive devices and gimmicks, are not the answer. You know this.

Since the beginning of Man, we've known how to go to sleep when sleep was what's next. Stories have been handed down by the village campfire, the fables of Aesop, Bible verses, and folklore, and comfort us in our journey toward sleep. And the ancient medicine and perhaps today's shaman offers holistic remedies to complement the effort.

This book will not, however, offer up any magic potions from the past, home remedies, or pharmaceutical solutions. Instead, the book focuses on using your mind power to train your brain to sleep.

Of course, any sleep disorder such as sleep apnea should be taken seriously and the prescribed therapeutic sleep equipment should be utilized. Sleep apnea impacts heart and brain functioning! When I suggest that one only needs the "sleep device between their ears" what I mean is that the crazy devices coming on the market today are just that — crazy, and costly, and in all likelihood, ineffective and unnecessary.

The really good news is, despite the distractions and pressures of daily life and stresses of the modern era, you do have the power within you to sleep well, and unless you have received an official medical diagnosis of chronic insomnia, the guidance offered in this book should help resolve your sleep issues. With a focus on your intentions and what you want to achieve (sleep), and a commitment to investing in your transformational shift, I am confident that you will do great! You do have much more control than you may realize in this moment. Embrace that notion as you proceed.

You can't cheat sleep, and you can't beat sleep. You were designed to spend one-third of your life on this planet in a deep, restful, and rejuvenating sleep. Embrace that fact.

As you begin reading, I want you to know that you can, indeed, sleep better than you do today, and you will begin to consistently sleep better and better, every night, and that the sleep eluding you now will soon come courting and become a natural part of your life once again.

I also want you to know that hypnosis — specifically, self-hypnosis — is the key, as you'll find in this book. You will learn enough to succeed with your sleep mastery and, who knows, it may spark further interest in hypnosis in general as a tool to improve other areas of your life as well.

Quite simply, by reading this book you will learn to master the art of falling asleep easily, without stress or anticipated difficulty, so that you can sleep with confidence to the point that it becomes natural once again! It is a book that helps you remove the struggle and the frustrations of trying to fall asleep. As Yoda says, "Do, or do not. There is no try." This is a book that helps you stop *trying* to sleep, and just *go* to sleep!

There will be a marvelous side effect to you sleeping well again. Imagine you with a broader smile, a better outlook on life, and more energy — enough to do the things you ought to do each day, and the things you want to do — all with more *joie de vivre* (i.e., joy for life) as the French would say. Isn't that the real goal for reading this book?

As you'll discover within these pages, it is possible to condition your mind and body to cooperate with your intentions, once you decide that sleep is what's to come next. Good sleep habits combined with self-hypnosis (which is simply a focused state of mind for the most part), along with a positive expectancy for the outcome you seek, will help you sleep better each night.

This book is *not* a book explaining why the world at large needs more sleep. There are many studies and scholarly articles on the subject. Nor is this a book that attempts to convince you to get more shut-eye, or how sleep affects the cell structure of the brain or other vital organs. You know that sleep is a part of life — about one-third of your time on this planet, in fact, as stated above. Finally, this is not a book about how much sleep you need at various stages of your life. Young people need more sleep than older people. We all need sleep when we are sick. You know how it feels when you are well-rested.

Can I let you in on a little secret? The key to sleeping well starts with teaching your mind and body how to relax. Yes, physical and mental relaxation are an important life skill. You'll learn enough to master your sleep skills, and then you'll become hooked on relaxation for life!

Even before that self-realization, the deeper secret to sleep success lies in having the right attitude about sleep and making sleep a priority. I expect that you will begin to notice, as you read on, that your beliefs and attitudes about sleep will shift. Thus, your journey to restful slumber will progress. It is all about your journey into sleep and being open to using self-hypnosis to get you there!

Let's keep this simple. Sleeplessness sucks, and you are on a journey to make sleeplessness a thing of your past, a non-issue. Commit to the journey!

Somewhere along the way, as life happened, you *unlearned* how to fall asleep. Stress, anxiety, fears, and a long list of emotional factors have crept in, making sleep more elusive. And the more you give chase, the more sleep tends to evade your pursuit.

Over the years, for whatever reasons, you let certain external factors or cues cause shifts in your sleep patterns and behaviors. The good news is that you can take back control of many external influencers affecting your sleep. As you delve deeper, on your journey toward sleep mastery, you'll learn how to relax your mind and body so that when it is time for sleep, you can enjoy a far better night's slumber than you are likely enjoying right now. In fact, as you condition your mind and body to sleep better — which will absolutely happen for you — you will begin to realize that you feel more energetic, with more stamina, more enthusiasm as you greet each day, and more *joie de vivre*, or zest for life. You will find that a new you will begin to emerge as you hone the art and skills of sleep once again, a new you filled with a desire to enjoy the day ahead. As you commit to the process of learning successful sleep strategies and habits, you begin to develop that truth, that awareness, which reveals the more you sleep, the more you get out of life. We need sleep to heal and rejuvenate.

The reverse is true, too. I venture to say that the *more fully you live your life each day*, the better you will sleep as well. Get and stay in the habit of living each day!

My Promise to You

I've written this book to help you sleep better! If you read and apply what you learn, you *will* sleep better. Embrace, if you will, the notion that you can discover how you can sleep better and end your chronic sleeplessness. You can do this holistically, using the power of your own mind, if you will only teach yourself, using this book as your guide.

The easy steps laid out for you in this book, once mastered by you, will change your life. What you will discover in the book comes from research and, more importantly, is directly based on professional clinical hypnosis work with thousands of clients and workshop attendees. And, you should know, I also use these techniques each night myself!

So, my promise to you is this: If you will simply trust the process of relearning to sleep, with the expectation that what you are learning in this book will work for you, better sleep is ahead. I promise.

Again, as stated earlier, if you are suffering from chronic insomnia, or suspect a physical concern such as sleep apnea may be causing your sleeplessness, please consult a bona fide medical doctor. Keep in mind that Doctor Google is not a real doctor! If you are using prescribed medications for sleep, I urge you to have a conversation with your doctor as well. I suggest that you do not turn to Doctor Google for a diagnosis of any suspected sleep disorder. Again, seek the advice and treatment from a qualified medical professional, and perhaps consult the International Classification of Sleep Disorders to help in your conversation with the doctor. Certainly, pursue a diagnosis, but know that stress is a major contributing factor, and a commitment to lower your stress will likely help you sleep better!

Take My Seven-Day "Fall Asleep Fast" Challenge

"A journey of a thousand miles begins with the first step."
—Lao Tzu

"But I have promises to keep,
And miles to go before I sleep,
And miles to go before I sleep."
—Robert Frost

Poetry teaches us so much. Your journey to sleep will be much shorter than Lao Tzu and Robert Frost might suggest, but it is a journey that only starts with your first step!

Your first step is to go to www.iamsleepingnow.com to get access to the additional resources I've developed for you.

There may likely be a part of you that is resisting sleep, for any of a variety of reasons. If this is the case with you — and you may not even realize it — then simply decide to stop seeking a solution, and let it *come* to you, stimulated by your increased awareness that sleep will come quite naturally if you let it!

Give yourself seven days of commitment to this holistic, natural approach and observe what happens. Who knows, it may be exactly what you have been seeking. You may even find yourself sleeping much better *tonight*, in fact, with no need to wait the full seven days to see results — and certainly no need to wait four weeks or ninety days, as others have suggested by using different methods. The I AM SLEEPING NOW method works fast!

Better sleep makes you more resilient and less stressed, free to enjoy a happier, more fulfilled day. If you are willing to choose to suspend judgment, stay open, and trust the process, this is going to be an easy effort, almost magical in fact.

Follow my seven days of sleep practice, as you increase your attention to your nightly snooze-o-rama. My seven-day challenge is quite easy. Simply decide to practice the sleep routine for seven days without judgment. This is a method, a way of conditioning your mind and body to sleep, driven by your intention, when you want to sleep.

It is my hope and expectation that you will begin to fall asleep more easily and more quickly tonight, simply because you are reading this book and pursuing a mind-based solution! As you will find described later in the book, please follow the seven-day sleep-conditioning exercises. By the seventh day or perhaps even sooner, you'll be sleeping better. When you embrace your sleep time as sacred time for you to heal your mind and body and soul, and you make it routine to practice the new habits of sleep, you are programming your mind for success!

In this book, I stress *acceptance* of your current sleeplessness as a first step, for whatever the reasons (which matter not at the moment), and then *inviting* sleep back into your life. Chasing sleep or trying to control insomnia is not going to work and only pushes it further away. In fact, be careful of labels and how they become affixed to your mind. If you continue to call yourself an insomniac, that label may not be a healthy choice if you are not diagnosed with a sleep disorder. Difficulty falling and staying asleep is often a symptom of stress, anxiety, fears, and worry. A sleep disorder is something altogether different and requires a medical diagnosis.

Heads-up!

While it is tempting to skim the book and skip to the I AM SLEEPING NOW method, I urge you to read every chapter. Let it unfold. There are gems in each chapter awaiting your discovery; pearls of wisdom, as they say.

My reader's challenge is this: Keep an open mind and apply what you are learning as you move through this book. Be patient with the process. Allow sleep to come to you. With optimism that you will master some new mind skills and true authenticity within yourself, and basic self-hypnosis skills learned in these pages, you will discover exactly what's been in the way of your sleeplessness.

Remember, also, that your sleep will improve as you bring your awareness and attention to your daily living. How you choose to start your day, no matter your circumstances, has a powerful impact on how your day ends. Please keep in mind that you can, indeed, program yourself to have a healthy outlook on life. It's important to your sleep mastery!

About the Journey

Chapters 1, 2, and 3 build the foundation for your long-term success.

Chapter 4 introduces you to the magic formula.

Chapters 5, 6, 7, and 8 help you take charge of your destiny.

Chapters 9, 10, and 11 explain the I AM SLEEPING NOW method.

Chapter 12 wraps it all up with final words of support.

If you want to enjoy intimacy even more, you'll love the 'bonus' chapter!

Remember, you can access the additional resources for this book at www.iamsleepingnow.com.

CONTENTS

INTRODUCTION

W elcome to your new journey toward masterful sleep. This is likely the road you've not yet taken. Be refreshed, and breathe a sigh of relief, for you are on the right path.

This sleep book is different and, in my opinion, long overdue. It's about sleep mastery, and learning how to de-hypnotize yourself from bad habits, reprogram your subconscious mind, and "relax into knowing" that, finally, you are on the path to your unique solution for preparing for and enjoying the restorative benefits of sleep. Hopefully, it will be my advice and not my writing that puts you to sleep!

I am on a mission, in fact, to put you, and the world, to sleep! Or, more accurately, to help the world to sleep better using quite natural skills and abilities by tapping into people's own mind power. It is so tempting, as a hypnotist, to ask you to imagine seeing a swinging watch and to recite to yourself, "I am getting sleepy." But I won't do that to you!

Here's a Zzz-Tip, right out of the gate. I know you are not sleeping well, or you would not be reading this book. But I want you to focus on the *present moment*, not your recent or long history of sleeplessness, nor even how you slept last night. I want you to embrace the truth that you are on a journey to find that elusive sleep secret and bring it back into your life, each night relaxing into the reality that what you learn and apply will make a huge difference for you physically, emotionally, mentally, and spiritually.

And, most importantly, I want you to acknowledge to yourself that shifting your mindset to present-moment living, while easier to talk about than to accomplish sometimes, is key to helping you take back control.

Let's face it. A good night's sleep is transformative, isn't it?

There's nothing like awakening feeling great and ready to greet the day with open arms. Who doesn't enjoy that feeling of bouncing out of bed, full of energy and anxious to get moving? Yet it eludes too many people.

As a professional hypnotist, I see clients who struggle with sleep issues, and it is a topic I have spoken widely about, having taught thousands of people to sleep easily and effortlessly once again. I have found that, unless they have a formal diagnosis of a sleep disorder, in most cases by focusing on reducing stress and anxiety and helping people to quiet their mind, they achieve what I call "sleep mastery." All without drugs, supplements, home remedies, contraptions and devices, or other inventions.

You already know that sleep is beneficial. It's mysterious, too, yet this is not a book about *why* we sleep. This mysterious realm where dreams live is essential to our health and well-being, our happiness in any given moment, and some of us will get so darned ornery and miserable without it. (Know somebody like that?) However, you need not understand the inner workings of a car's engine to drive it, and to realize that you need to properly maintain it if you want the vehicle to perform reliably. Similarly, the same applies for sleep; you need not know all of the inner neuroscience of sleep in order to sleep soundly. You do, however, need to get proper sleep for you to perform well! It's safe to say you know that already, but let me make a point...

Sleep is the invisible X-factor. And self-hypnosis unlocks the mind. Sleep is well recognized as a game-changer by professionals in all walks of life:

- Business leaders know that a workforce that sleeps well and comes to their position well-rested and refreshed creates certain advantages in a competitive environment, simply improving overall quality of their products and services. Workforce accidents are lower, job performance is better, absenteeism is reduced, and wellness statistics are improved.

- Athletes and sports teams at all levels recognize the importance of sleep for achieving peak performance. Skills, talents, and abilities are essential, but the team or individual that shows up refreshed and ready brings an advantage.
- All branches of the military now view sleep as a force multiplier. It's taught in all service academies, and senior command officers prioritize sleep in field or mission readiness.
- College students and professionals studying for advancement know that sleep is essential for academic performance.

This is a book that helps you take back control of what I call your *habitual rituals* — or your tiny success habits regarding sleeping — and to guide you in making small, incremental habit changes which, as success builds, gives you more confidence in your ability to enjoy a good night's sleep.

Aside from enjoying a rejuvenating and recharging rest, as well as a chance for cells to repair and reconnect, scientific research is showing that improved sleep positively affects our ability for memory recall, and it enhances our learning and skills development. From the boardroom to the bedroom, your sleep health matters.

As for myself, sleep first became an issue for me as a young sailor in the U.S. Navy's Submarine Service, a long time ago. Being new to the boat I was assigned to, I didn't get my own bunk for about three months. In the meantime, I slept on a makeshift bunk atop two ominous nuclear war-tipped torpedoes, called SUBROCs. If I can learn to sleep lying on a 250-kiloton nuclear depth charge, I think that you can program yourself to sleep like a baby in your bed, using my hypnotic sleeping method.

Imagine sleeping between two torpedoes, in a noisy space, lights always on, and people always walking past you, some more aware than others. If a sub sailor can sleep in these conditions, you will master your sleep skills in your own bed!

Anyway, at that time, in the 1970s, life at sea aboard a nuclear submarine was scheduled by an 18-hour day, not the traditional 24-hour cycle that the rest of the world follows. It played havoc on the body clock. It was a challenge on the body and the circadian rhythm, and the only light came from a fluorescent bulb! Imagine six hours on watch, followed by twelve hours off watch, which was time for sleep and other tasks you could not perform while on watch (it could have been department-related duties, or training and ship's drills, or time to catch the movie of the day in the ship's galley, or even do laundry and take a traditional three-minute shower when we had extra water). We literally did not know what day it was sometimes, unless we kept track, because we did not have the sun, stars, and the moon to tell us the hour of the day. Our body clock was seriously confused while at sea.

Then, sometime in 2014 or thereabouts, the Navy changed to the 24-hour day, to the elation of sailors and the command staff. Instead of 6 and 12, it became 8-on and 16-off watch cycles. The 24-hour day was back, and everyone loved it. According to the *Navy Times* magazine, "It has had an extraordinary impact on a couple of areas. First, mission execution and alertness. And on the eight-hour schedule, nobody fell asleep as the contact manager standing up. The officer of the deck wasn't leaning up against the periscope with both eyes closed and being slapped by the junior officer of the deck to stay awake, as was once common. The second part is it dramatically improves morale on the ship."

I was a civilian long before the Navy made this important shift to the 24-hour day for submariners. Back when I served, while I don't believe our mission ever suffered, I often did wonder where we found the energy and stamina to do all that we did, deep under the ocean's waves. We had seemed to be tired a lot, grabbing naps and a good night's sleep along the way. But perhaps yesterday's sub sailors were tougher. A subject for another book, perhaps. Someday.

I also recall one particular sleep-deprived, mission-critical task that kept me awake for a full 58 hours. Tied up along the pier in Pusan, South Korea, the entire submarine crew was waiting on me to rewire the inertial navigation system so we could get back underway and on patrol in the Sea of Japan. Due to my job specialization, I was the only person available for the task (along with the assistance of a couple others in the division). It was no fun. Lots of coffee and support, and the Commanding Officer breathing down my neck, and a few short naps when I could steal them. As difficult as it was at the time, it proved essential, as that repair allowed us to sneak through the Tsugaru Straits between Honshu and Hokkaido a few days later. I think I was asleep for that transit. When passing through the straits, it was the inertial navigation system that accurately guided us, undetected, in relatively shallow waters.

Why is this relevant?

Well, I share the above only because, as you know, sleep is essential for all. We all have unique demands that impact our quality and quantity of sleep. And, most importantly, I want you to know that sleep is no longer elusive for you! This book presents some very easy and powerful techniques used by the military, by business leaders, and by normal everyday people just like you! And, my Tsugaru Straits experience can be a metaphor for yourself, when you have to believe in yourself, and muster the energy to get the job done.

Now it's your turn to master the art of sleeping when your intention is such.

Since you are reading this book, here with me now... let me say that it is time for you to stop *trying* to fall asleep, and simply *fall* asleep — and also stay asleep longer. Sleep becomes elusive when you seek it too aggressively, so shift that whole effort, and instead let it come to you.

These four magic words, "I AM SLEEPING NOW," will help you easily and intentionally enter the realm of a healing, restful sleep. Throughout my years as a professional hypnotist, I have been teaching people how to take back control of their thoughts, emotions, and behaviors when it is time to fall asleep, using the phrase "I am sleeping now." It is magical — and it works!

This book is all about teaching you how to put your mind and body in a sleep state. It is not an academic book about the science of sleep. It is about your intentional, *conscious intervention* and desire to sleep — a pattern interrupt, driven by your quest to feel better when you arise from sleep.

It is about you intervening and, as I said, interrupting your thoughts to change the trajectory, calm the mind, and end the cycle of sleeplessness and its consequences. Low energy and a sluggish start lead to an unending struggle to sleep better, which in turn leads to more worry and stress over sleep, resulting in poor quality sleep, and thus the cycle continues. Diet, mental health, and even spiritual health suffer as well.

No matter your profession or circumstances in life, you need to master the art of sleep so you can be more fully present in your waking state. Besides, sleeping better leads to longevity in your years!

It's imperative that you find relief from your sleeplessness *fast*. It's also imperative that you relearn how to sleep without habitual medications (a decision you'll make with your doctor, please). This book is designed to help you do this, and to help you to sleep like a baby once again. That is what you want, correct?

Think about it.

You used to sleep like a baby. Remember? Can you pretend you remember? Just like a baby you observe today, who can fall asleep at the drop of a hat, you can train your mind and body to fall easily and effortlessly asleep when you want to do so. Whether for a good night's restful slumber, a short nap, or even a brief hypnotic recharge, you can learn to clear your mind and focus on entering the realm of sleep *on command.*

And you can do so, likely, without the need for medications and homeopathy or strange brews! Of course, you will have to discuss that with your doctor. This book is not about diagnosing or treating a physical sleep disorder, as I have made clear. But sleep is, indeed, big business, as I have hinted. Researchers are slicing and dicing the industry, and the investment opportunities, so that manufacturers and venture capitalists can bring new sleep aids to your pillow, and your money to their mattress!

Since the beginning of mankind, we've been sleeping just fine. Yes, the occasional flood, war, saber-toothed tiger at the cave entrance, and natural disasters kept us from slumber. But I want you to embrace that inner natural ability to sleep well again by controlling your stress, anxiety, habits, and how you respond to what is going on in the world around you. You have more control than you might realize or want to admit.

Know this, too. Sleep medications may provide short-term relief (if in fact any at all). They are not intended for long-term use. In my practice, I help more people than I want to count to stop taking sleep meds that were negatively impacting their life. It baffles me why so many in the medical profession prescribe sleep meds when they know that upwards of ninety percent of patients present stress and anxiety symptoms. It's like an auto mechanic telling a customer that an oil change and a radiator flush will fix their brake issue.

Non-pharmaceutical solutions are seldom presented by the medical community. You present a symptom; they present a pill. No sleep medication in the world will help you solve or alleviate the angst you are feeling, caused by your emotional state. Improving your sleep requires an inner journey of reflection and perhaps conscious intervention to change a few things. Pills cannot do that, but they are an alternative for those who won't face reality.

I am not a doctor, and I don't try to play one on the internet. I do feel, however, that primary care physicians would be doing better for their patients by ordering a sleep study, along with therapy or clinical hypnosis, before prescribing habit-forming drugs for sleep issues mostly caused by emotional discord. Fortunately, I see more and more patients who are advocating for themselves and refusing the sleep meds as they seek a holistic solution.

I should also point out that sleeplessness is an epidemic — a pandemic, actually, according to the CDC. Sleep deprivation is considered a serious public health crisis. I could cite a million sources that will tell you that you, and the rest of the world's citizens, are likely not getting enough sleep. But I will refrain. You know that you are not getting enough quality sleep and you do not need a university or medical school to tell you so!

As a professional hypnotist, I have spoken widely to all age groups about falling asleep using hypnosis, and I've taught thousands of people to harness the power of their subconscious mind to help them with their intention of once again enjoying a good night's sleep. Like others I have helped, I am assuming that somewhere along the way, you conditioned yourself to struggle with sleep. Struggle no more.

So, with your goal of mastering the skills of a sound sleeper, let's proceed.

Plan to sleep better tonight, and to begin to hone your "fall asleep" skills as you condition your mind and body to welcome and embrace your desire to sleep — and garner the full cooperation of every cell, every muscle, every part of yourself!

Let's get started.

Indulge me for a moment. I want you to imagine that every cell in your body is smiling at you from the inside. You see, they know the power of your intention. They are happy that you are open to the whole concept of mind/body communication. They are happy you are doing this! Your cells are anticipating a return to health, and an opportunity to repair, rejuvenate, and revitalize their cellular health. They are anticipating a return to the old you, who is a new you, once again enjoying the benefits of a good night's sleep.

Imagine that your mind and body are excited to know — all due to your intentions to pursue a fast and powerful, natural sleep solution — that your restorative powers will make you feel more vibrant, and more energized for your day ahead, with a renewed optimism!

You will sleep well again, so that you may live well again!

Isn't that the ultimate goal? Sleeping better to function better, and thus live a better, happier life. Imagine it, because that is your journey here in these pages.

Sleep is at your doorstep and will come in if you invite it. One of the keys to enjoying better sleep is learning how to live more so in the present moment, in the here and now, rather than living in the past (with regret, perhaps), or living in the future in a state of worry and anxiety.

This book will give you some of the tools to focus on present-moment living.

As the National Sleep Foundation tells us, "How we live our lives directly impacts how we sleep. From how much coffee we drink in the morning to our bedtime routine at night, the right lifestyle choices can mean the difference between a good and a bad night of sleep."

Sleep health encompasses four primary areas, some of which we'll touch on, others are for your exploration with your doctor, all of which factor into your success:

- Age Factors: How much sleep is enough?
- The Bedroom: The environment matters!
- Lifestyle: Foods, exercise, napping, sex, coffee?
- Science: Melatonin, lighting, essential oils, supplements, technology?

We may *touch upon* some of the sage advice within these four areas, but the primary purpose of the book is to help you easily and quickly fall and fall back asleep using a proven method that I call I AM SLEEPING NOW.

There is a fifth area I would like to offer to you as well: How you live your life — your character, values, and beliefs — all matter. You will get the best sleep when you hit the pillow with a clear conscience, knowing that the day was fruitful, productive, or simply peaceful. Tending to a healthy mind, body, and spirit during the day helps us to sleep better each night. All this aside, however, the method you will learn in this book will help you fall asleep more quickly, and also to get back to sleep more quickly should you awaken during the night.

You will find, as this book unfolds, that you will begin to feel better knowing you can *take greater and greater control* of the situation, using your mind and your resolve to sleep better again, as you teach yourself how to do what used to come so naturally!

Can you really train your mind and body to easily fall asleep?

Can you quiet your mind and stop the racing thoughts that seem to come from nowhere, using the power of your intention to become more calm, more relaxed, and so internally peaceful that you slip into a slumber?

The answer is a resounding "Yes!"

In fact, you will find that sleeping is once again so easy, you'll be doing it with your eyes closed! Pun intended. Bear with the humor.

Calming the mind will calm the body. Calming the heart and brain will calm the mind.

One more thing. This is important.

There are many books that discuss *why* we sleep. This book, as you know, is about *how* to fall and stay asleep — without medications or any other types of sleep aids.

You might be the type of person who reads this entire book from cover to cover, absorbing and applying as you go, improving your sleep practice each night. Or you might be the type of person who reads this book to help fall asleep, and finds the head starts a-bobbing as you try to turn the pages. That's okay! Let the pages and your eyelids become heavy. That's right. You are doing great! Try to stay with me, as sleep beckons.

Whether the process of reading my book does the trick for you, or if the I AM SLEEPING method you are learning is more reliable, the result is the same. You'll fall asleep quickly and easily! Hopefully, it's not my writing that causes you to drift off, but if so, we can still claim victory!

One more important perspective on this topic. It is time for you to unconditionally love and accept yourself and practice a little mindful self-compassion by deciding to grant yourself the gift of sound, peaceful, stress-free, and restful sleep each night.

CHAPTER ONE

Sleep Is at Your Doorstep, Ringing the Bell – Go Open the Door and Let It In!

"I love sleep. My life has the tendency to fall apart when I'm awake, you know?"

—Ernest Hemingway, American author

The chapter title is an allusion to the great song from Paul McCartney and Wings, "Let 'Em In." It was a smash hit from their album *Wings at the Speed of Sound* in the 1970s.

I won't cite the lyrics here for copyright reasons, but the message should come through clear enough: Do yourself a favor when sleep is knocking at your door — welcome it, and let it in!

Sounds simple enough, right? When you "open the door," so to speak, and let sleep in, you'll be off to dreamland at the speed of sound! Yet, before you answer the door to let sleep in, let us do *this* first. Before we go any further, let's start out by visiting some of the reasons we might struggle to fall asleep, stay asleep, or sleep more deeply:

- Stress and anxiety
- Fears and emotions
- Loneliness
- Grief and sadness
- Inability to forgive oneself or others
- Self-imposed pressure
  - Perfection
  - Achievement

- o Type-A personalities
- Unresolved conflict
- Regrets
- Loss of hope
- Negative self-talk
- Finances
- Relationship issues

There are countless other reasons that are unique to you, and many more that are commonly held. As we move through the book, we'll talk about ways to set the nagging issues aside so that sleep can come to you when summoned.

So, please invite Hypnos, the god of sleep, into your world.

I'll not delve into Greek and Roman mythology here (you can thank me later) but suffice it to say that Hypnos, the ancient Greek god of sleep — and for whom hypnosis was named — can help bring about the sleep you desire. All you need to do is declare it to make it so, much like when Dorothy says her famous line, "There's no place like home," in *The Wizard of Oz*! You'll see.

If you could travel back in time for a brief consultation with Hypnos, or if you could bring him here to your present moment, I wonder what wisdom he would impart? Imagine channeling him right now. Yes, you've got a few minutes with the God of Sleep himself!

So, I wonder what you'd ask Hypnos if you could summon him now and were granted a personal consultation? Would you ask him:

- *Why can I not fall asleep?*
- *What is it that is keeping me from enjoying a good night's sleep?*
- *What do I need to change in my life so that sleep comes more easily?*
- *What is the secret to falling asleep?*
- *What is it that keeps me awake in the middle of the night?*
- *Do I need to start or stop any habits that are keeping sleep away?*

All great questions! You can imagine to yourself what his responses might be. In addition, he'd likely say that you need to lower the arousal of your sympathetic nervous system and your parasympathetic nervous system (learn to relax), and:

- Deal with the stresses in your life to avoid them becoming an overwhelming cause of distress.
- Live in the present moment, learning from the past, with an eye on tomorrow yet grateful for your gifts and blessings.
- Master relaxation as a natural tool (or weapon) for combatting maladaptive responses — specifically, that you learn progressive muscle relaxation.
- Prioritize and revere sleep.
- Show yourself that you love yourself by embracing changes to help you sleep.
- Learn to become more resilient in dealing with the challenges of life.

Zzz-Tip: In other words, he would say that you must learn to relax, and to enjoy the therapeutic mind and body benefits that come with a relaxed mind and body.

We all know that sleep is a basic human need, and it supports healthy brain function. And, it works to maintain our physical health, repairing cellular issues in the rest state. It's a time-out for our mind and body connection to do the magic it was designed to perform. Sleep strengthens our immune system; it is a master regulator of our health and well-being.

I wonder if you can remember a time when sleep came so naturally? Perhaps in your crib, or after an afternoon learning how to walk. Or maybe after a training session learning how to ride your bicycle? Back then, you were good at crashing just about anywhere. (And by "crashing," I don't mean your bicycle!)

Yes, and then the pressures of life started disrupting sleep. Over time, stress and anxiety, fears and emotions, loneliness, unresolved conflict, finances, relationships, and a variety of self-imposed ideas started to rule your life.

It's time for you to take back control.

Imagine getting back to enjoying that feeling of falling asleep, with stress-free effort, if there's effort at all, and simply letting your mind and body rejuvenate while you rest.

That's where we're going with this book!

Every being on the planet needs sleep, man and beast alike. And when we humans do not get our sleep, we can become quite beastly. So, you see, family, friends, and co-workers alike will celebrate your return to sleeping success.

We all know that sleep is important. Quality sleep, and enough of it each night, is essential to our health and well-being. Our brain requires it, and, in fact, our entire body needs sleep. Our brain functions better, and cells communicate better. Sleep is essential. You knew that!

It is important to keep in mind that sleeping is a natural state that *restores* energy spent during the day, it also *replenishes* and *rejuvenates* the immune, nervous, skeletal, and muscular systems. Sleep keeps the brain working and is thereby vital to healthy brain function, physical health, and emotional well-being.

Sleeplessness can result in:

- Lower levels of energy
- Hormonal imbalance
- Increased stress and anxiety levels
- Loss of concentration or focus
- Unsteady mood such as being angry, sad, depressed, impatient, etc.
- Hindrance in cognitive performance creating an inability to make decisions, solve problems, control emotions and behaviors, or cope with change
- Health conditions such as high blood pressure, heart disease, stroke, obesity

As you begin to sleep better, you'll be lessening the impact of these issues or avoiding them altogether!

As the National Institutes of Health (NIH) says:

In fact, your brain and body stay remarkably active while you sleep. Recent findings suggest that sleep plays a housekeeping role that removes toxins in your brain that build up while you are awake. Everyone needs sleep, but its biological purpose remains a mystery. Sleep affects almost every type of tissue and system in the body — from the brain, heart, and lungs to metabolism, immune function, mood, and disease resistance. Research shows that a chronic lack of sleep, or getting poor quality sleep, increases the risk of disorders including high blood pressure, cardiovascular disease, diabetes, depression, and obesity. Sleep is a complex and dynamic process that affects how you function in ways scientists are now beginning to understand.

That is about as scientific as we'll get in this book on the topic of sleep science.

Our focus lies in teaching you the easy-to-master sleep skills so that you can get back to enjoying a good night's sleep each night! After all, as previously mentioned in the Introduction, you don't need to study the mechanics of a car engine in order to drive a vehicle. You do, however, need to know proper maintenance tips and driving skills.

Well, the same is true for learning how to sleep well. You need to master the skills.

Restless, sleepless nights are no fun. We all need and deserve a good night's sleep. Our body and mind require sleep to grow, rest, and rejuvenate. Sleep repairs the body, and it is essential to our health! Now, with that brilliant observation out of the way, let's start this journey toward your good night's sleep. While there is no need to state the obvious or to present a dissertation on the science of sleep, you may find a few scholarly references in this book, as needed to support the discussion. Fair enough?

The goal here is to help you sleep using the power of your mind to do so. There are plenty of other books on the topic of sleep science. You and I know sleep is important to the quality of life we enjoy, and to our health.

I have written this book from the heart. I want you to sleep well! It is my goal for you, but it must become yours if you think it makes sense for you, and that includes doing the work that invites sleepiness when sleep is what's next. You should be able to get a good night's sleep without drugs of any kind, be it pharmaceutical or alternative solutions such as melatonin, or other (supposedly) short-term supplements or medications. If you are taking prescription medications for sleep aids, have a conversation with your doctor and decide whether you should be weaned off these harmful medications. While this book does not present medical advice, it is always wise to periodically review the need for your medications. Keep in mind that in regard to sleeplessness, any prescribed medications should be considered a short-term treatment of the symptoms.

Getting to the root causes of your sleeplessness is crucial, yet this is generally not something your primary care doctor has either the time to explore or the time and skills to address. If they did, then medical professionals would advise you to lower your stress levels, get more exercise, and change a few unhealthy habits, among other things. Sometimes they do. But more often than not, they do not tell you how to make changes, and while for the most part they mean well, usually they will just end up merely prescribing medications. Unfortunately, it's what they were trained to do; it's called Western medicine. They might also refer you to a sleep clinic to determine whether you have a diagnosable sleep disorder such as sleep apnea, restless leg syndrome, narcolepsy, circadian rhythm sleep-wake disorder, or any of the others as defined in the DSM-5 "Sleep Disorders" section. The DSM-5, or *Diagnostic and Statistical Manual of Mental Disorders*, defines ten different types of sleep disorders, none of which are addressed in *this* book.

On this topic, if you believe you have a sleep disorder or a mental health issue, please get a medical diagnosis. Internet research for a self-diagnosis or listening to big pharma commercials for sleep medicines may yield a clue, for exploration with your doctor. Are you forming a self-diagnosis based on what you are reading? Be careful to not adopt the symptoms you read online. You could talk yourself into developing the symptoms! Yes, it's great to self-advocate and do some research but be careful about labeling yourself as having a disorder or a syndrome when your sleep problems may simply be rooted in stress and anxiety about life. As you will see repeated elsewhere as this book unfolds, see your doctor if you are struggling with sleep issues that you may feel need a diagnosis.

You might feel that falling asleep can *seem* so complex, or worse, frustrating, and so elusive. I can understand that perspective because I see far too many clients who make it complex! But falling asleep and staying asleep is actually pretty easy, once you relearn the skills you once mastered and begin to reprogram yourself!

As we begin this journey toward better sleep, remember that it is not at all unusual to toss and turn and suffer through a seemingly restless night. It is something many of us experience. Things happen in life and sometimes our minds just do not want to settle down. The good news is, as you embrace this very simple strategy using the four magic words "I AM SLEEPING NOW," you will learn the physical and mental discipline through practice and conditioning which will allow you to sleep when you have that intention.

Let's face it. People who can't sleep are very tired. Tired of taking advice from well-intended people who magically and effortlessly seem to enjoy a good night's sleep and brag about it!

Am I right?

Most of the people I help are also quite tired of sleep medications, and tired of all of the various remedies and pill concoctions touted on social media by their fellow sleep sufferers claiming success. The people I speak with have tried everything, including consulting the internet, taking "expert advice" from insomniacs in online support groups, and from well-meaning friends.

Am I wrong?

Well, it's time for something completely different! I contend that too many of the sleepless who spend their life on Facebook commiserating in insomnia groups are just looking to share their misery, or sell their own audio recordings or unproven sleep products.

As an aside, I feel it's important here to differentiate between a diagnosed sleep disorder causing insomnia, and acute or chronic sleeplessness that can lead to a sleep disorder. It may sound like a very fine point of distinction. Perhaps. But I want you to know that you can take control of your sleeplessness, in very many cases, by making some simple, incremental habit changes to lower stress and anxiety, and by adjusting a few other dynamics.

As described on www.webmd.com:

> Insomnia is a sleep disorder in which you have trouble falling and/or staying asleep. The condition can be short-term (acute) or can last a long time (chronic). It may also come and go. Acute insomnia lasts from 1 night to a few weeks. Insomnia is chronic when it happens at least 3 nights a week for 3 months or more.
>
> There are two types of insomnia: primary and secondary.
>
> - *Primary insomnia*: This means your sleep problems are not linked to any other health condition or problem.
> - *Secondary insomnia*: This means you have trouble sleeping because of a (physical or mental) health condition or possible substance use/abuse issue.

In addressing your individual, unique situation, I'll bet that very few people in your world have suggested *self-hypnosis* to help you fall asleep, stay asleep, and wake refreshed! Doctors, friends and family, and others, simply have not discovered the benefits of self-hypnosis, especially when it comes to sleeping better!

We'll explore the particulars of this in greater detail later on. But, right now, for the fun of it… please pause to practice this exercise just once or twice:

Take a moment now… get comfortable where you are seated… I

*invite you right now to take in a slow and comfortable deep breath...
get comfortable where you are... and simply breathe in through your
nose... hold it for the count of 4 or 5... exhale comfortably and
now... focus on the exchange of oxygen and carbon dioxide as your
heart and lungs work together for your highest and best... I would
like you to count down slowly, from 5... Down to 4... 3... relaxing...
2... and 1... As you breathe and continue to relax... say I AM SLEEP-
ING NOW... another relaxing breath... Repeat 10 times... with a
calm, slow relaxing breath between each count... and get to the number 10... if you can!*

Did you pause from reading to do it? It feels good to feel good
knowing you have this inner natural talent! Are you noticing that
you feel a little better, a little more relaxed? It's a great, well-
proven exercise in mind and body working together driven by intention.

I hope you paused to practice the above, because every day and
in every way, you will be better and better at taking back control
using your breath to aid you. There is certainly more to discuss,
and we'll get to it further on. I want you to begin to discover the
hypnotic concepts behind this simple present-tense sleeping
command: *"I am sleeping now."*

First, I want you to realize that, whether you are aware of it or
not, you are frequently in a light trance. We are *always* in a trance,
all of us, numerous different types of trances, in fact, throughout
the day. This could be the subject of another book in itself! But the
idea of trance utilization is what is important here.

Ever notice while driving that you arrived at your highway
exit wondering how you got there? Your mind and body were
driving the car while your conscious mind was off daydreaming
somewhere. Ever been so focused on a project or task that you lost
track of time or what was going on around you? Same thing.

Back to you getting a good night's sleep tonight!

When it's time to go to bed to sleep, then it's time to shift your
trance to the *sleep* trance. I'll show you how later, even though
the four magic words you've already learned are really all you

need, plus a little preparation. (There is only one other reason to go to bed, by the way, and that is sex. Your bed is *not* the place to eat breakfast, play on your phone, go on Facebook, text your friend, or attend a video conference. Comprende? Your bedroom is for two purposes only.)

Self-accountability is key here. The primary reason you struggle with sleep is because of habits, choices, and stress and anxiety that keep your mind in overdrive. You must acknowledge your current habits as you master your sleep skills and decide which ones you will address and change for the better!

To get to the sleep state, one must pass through the hypnotic state of mind (in other words, since our brainwaves are slowest during sleep, and being in the hypnotic state is that sleep-like just-before-sleep state). So, doesn't it make sense to use self-hypnosis to bring you closer to sleep? Yes, absolutely!

Let's talk about brainwaves for a moment, in order to help understand the journey to and from the sleep state. (I promised to limit the science of sleep within these pages. But allow me to touch upon this for just a bit, if you will, and I'll try not to get too overly technical here.) In the clinical hypnosis process, we utilize hypnosis as a tool to offer suggestions for the subconscious mind to consider and apply. Using self-hypnosis, you will be, quite literally, as a direct result of your intended fall-asleep process, guiding yourself to the sleep state. In this book, you will learn techniques that bring you to the brainwave states that foster relaxation and calmness, that stimulate focus and creativity, and enable restful sleep. In other words, you will learn how to bring yourself to a nice hypnotic state for all the benefits to be enjoyed there, and to pass through that hypnagogic state and continue with an intentional transition to the sleep state!

According to *Scientific American*, December 22, 1997:

> There are four brainwave states that range from the high amplitude, low frequency delta to the low amplitude, high frequency beta. These brainwave states range from deep dreamless sleep to high arousal. The same four brainwave states are common to the human species. Men, women and

children of all ages experience the same characteristic brainwaves. They are consistent across cultures and country boundaries. When we go to bed and read for a few minutes before attempting sleep, we are likely to be in low beta. When we put the book down, turn off the lights and close our eyes, our brainwaves will descend from beta, to alpha, to theta, and finally, when we fall asleep, to delta.

When you are journeying toward sleep, you are passing from beta, to alpha, to theta, and to delta — where sleep happens! We use hypnosis and relaxation techniques to move into alpha, which enables clear visualization, contemplating, and meditating. The I AM SLEEPING NOW method to program yourself for better sleep starts with a journey to the alpha state. Getting there is easy. Calm relaxed breathing will do it, and it's an essential practice in your soon-to-be new pre-sleep routine. It jumpstarts the process!

Brain Waves Chart

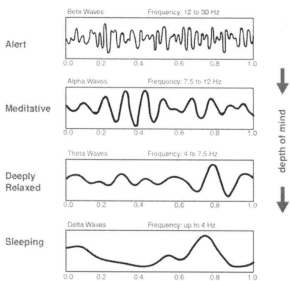

The process of trying to go to sleep is a beta state effort. Deciding to stop trying, and receive sleep, first as an image — a self-fulfilling prophecy — is much better, and requires that shift into alpha. Even Yoda, in his wisdom ("Do, or do not. There is no try"), was encouraging a move to the hypnotic state!

Theta is the next state, where the brainwaves slow further, allowing for, as is evidence-based, a deeper state of receptivity to suggestions. So, visualize you, relaxing deeper, and as you go, feeding yourself this suggestion: "I Am Sleeping Now," almost whispering it to yourself as you drift off to sleep, right into delta!

So, what I'd like you to know about brainwaves, quite simply, is that they slow down when we enter a relaxed, calm state, and they slow down even further when we slip into a good night's slumber (or even a short nap). And, in the alpha or theta state, your mind is more readily open to embracing and applying new ideas that support one's intentions and goals. You'll discover that self-hypnosis can take you to the theta state for 15–20 minutes, giving you the equivalent benefit of a one-hour nap! While in the alpha or theta brainwave state, your mind is open and receptive to new suggestions, that you allow into your mind to embrace and consider, and then apply! Any additional discussion right now would start to take us off course, so I won't elaborate any further. As I've said, you do not need to know the idiosyncrasies of a car's engine to drive it. Same is true here, although I do invite you to explore hypnosis as a tool for better living!

If you are tossing and turning and unable to sleep, it may be the ruminations you are entertaining in a beta brainwave state. The good news is that you can (and you are) able to take control of your mind and body and descend into theta and delta on command!

Please keep in mind my goal for you, in writing this book. It is intended to help you invite sleep back into your life. All I ask you to do is to keep an open mind, setting all judgment and negative self-talk aside as you proceed on this easy journey, and to commit to read this entire book and to practice each night for a week. You are on a journey to finally tackle this problem and, as you enjoy success, you will likely soon start teaching others how to conquer sleep issues as you master it for yourself!

It requires belief, visualization, mental rehearsal, discipline, and determination — all to be discussed in this book, and each element easily mastered — if this is what you want for yourself.

You see, your mind is a very powerful resource. Your subconscious mind knows your *true intentions* and beliefs and seeks to align your mind so it can do its job for you! Our subconscious mind assists us in so many ways, including protecting us and serving us by off-loading and taking on certain jobs from our conscious mind. One of those jobs it wants to do for you is to calm your mind and body so you can enjoy a restorative and rejuvenating night's sleep. Of course, you must do your part as well for this sleep mastery to be possible.

So, to recap the big picture, the goal here is to start getting a better night's sleep so that you can consistently sleep well. Getting a good night's sleep becomes your expected outcome, with the expectation and the anticipation that you will begin to awaken each day more refreshed and ready to face the new day ahead.

As a professional hypnotist for the past thirteen years, I have helped thousands of people to sleep better, using easy-to-learn self-hypnosis techniques that quiet the mind and allow for sleep to arrive.

Now it's your turn.

Again, keep an open mind toward becoming more empowered, and begin to see yourself taking back control of this issue once and for all.

Let's begin by focusing on what you *do* want, as opposed to what you do *not* want, because, as we say in my profession, where the attention goes, the energy flows.

What we think about becomes real.

Picture yourself on this path toward sleep mastery and know that you are moving in this direction. Get ready to sleep like a professional. If counting sheep works for you, keep counting. If not, then keep reading!

Since before the word hypnosis was coined, people have often struggled to consistently get a good night's sleep. Sometimes that sleeplessness has been short-lived, while other times it may last for years. The truth is that throughout mankind's existence, in our constant pursuit of sleep, we've found it to be frequently elusive. And it seems the more we chase it, the harder it becomes.

Keep in mind that, although people have struggled with sleep throughout the ages, the world has changed. Prior to the industrial age, farmers arose late at night to feed or milk their cows, then went back to sleep until the rooster crowed. (Today's farmers still have interrupted sleep!) Then, as people left the farm for factory jobs there was no need to arise in the dark of night. In today's modern world, we have a 24-hour news cycle, internet access around the globe, and far too many distractions that keep us awake.

As I said at the top of this chapter, sleep *is* at your doorstep, ringing the doorbell. Answer the door and invite it in, as Paul McCartney would likely advise, right? In fact, while you are at it, serve up a cup of green tea or chamomile tea in the evening. Mindfully enjoying a cup of tea an hour before bed may bring surprising, relaxing, peaceful, and harmonious results. As I tell my clients, and as I've already stated previously but emphasize here once again, *stop chasing* sleep and let it come to you instead.

I'll also share an observation now that many, in most cases, do not like to hear — that sleeplessness comes from *self-created* bad habits. This will all be discussed further as we go along. Yet be aware, you have some decisions and choices ahead of you as we move to sleep mastery. Getting a consistent good night's sleep also means that dealing with stress, anxiety, fears, and emotional issues are all part of the solution. The good news here, again, is that hypnosis is a great tool for taking back control of the awake stages of your daily life! A large part of your success will come from a serious look at current habits, and then putting a hypnotic plan in place to end or change them, clearing the way of obstacles that may hinder better sleep.

On a biological cellular level, sleep repairs our body. Lack of sleep affects different parts of the brain differently. Although this book is not about the science of sleep, it is important to know that sleep is restorative. Up until the last half of the previous century, most people believed sleep was a passive activity during which the body and brain did nothing much at all. "But it turns out that sleep is a period during which the brain is engaged in a number of activities necessary to life — which are closely linked to *quality* of life," notes Johns Hopkins neurologist and sleep expert Mark Nan Wu, M.D., Ph.D.

Making sense of this on a practical level, one key to your sleep success is to prioritize and respect sleep as a vitally important part of life and of your quality of daily living.

A Word About Insomnia: Get a Professional Diagnosis

Insomnia is defined as a sleep disorder in which a person has persistent problems falling or staying asleep. It is well documented that most cases of insomnia are related to poor sleep habits, depression, anxiety, lack of exercise, chronic illness, or certain medications.

Symptoms of insomnia may include difficulty falling or staying asleep, and not feeling very well rested. Many people struggle to get a good night's sleep. They experience a variety of problems with sleeping including not getting sufficient sleep, poor quality of sleep, not feeling well-rested when they awaken, and restless sleep. Sleep problems can cause fatigue and difficulties functioning throughout the day, affecting the quality of life. Insomnia can be short-term or can last a long time.

Insomnia is complex. As a clinical hypnotist who works with many clients struggling to sleep better, I've become aware of a large number of people who announce they have a diagnosed sleeping disorder such as insomnia, yet many with no diagnosis other than their own internet research. They accept their own Google diagnosis, assume symptoms, and *voilà*! Self-labeled, self-diagnosed insomniacs. Foolish and unwise to say the least. Most of the time these people's issues stem from unmanaged stress and anxiety. Some believe that only medications will solve their

25

issues, while others will seek to avoid sleep medications. As you explore your own situation, be very wary and very vigilant about sleep medications, their effects on your mind and body, and the possibility for addiction.

If your doctor rules out any physical issues or an official medical diagnosis of insomnia is not provided, there is a very good chance that the techniques in this book will work just fine. All you need is a personal commitment to allow sleep to come, an open mind, and some practice.

Insomnia is both well-studied and a mystery all at once. As Haynes, Follingstad, and McGowan surmised in their scholarly article "Insomnia: Sleep patterns and anxiety level," published in the *Journal of Psychosomatic Research* (vol. 18, pp 69–74, 1974):

> Insomniacs typically report that it requires an excessive length of time to fall asleep once they are in bed and/or that they awaken frequently during the night. There are, however, no established criteria for differentiating insomniacs from non-insomniacs … [It has been] suggested that a high level of autonomic arousal may be a concomitant, if not causal, factor in abnormal sleep patterns. Because sleep is associated with low levels of autonomic arousal, individuals who are highly aroused may have trouble in falling asleep or may awaken frequently at night.

They went on to say in their report:

> [E]lectromyography (EMG) levels, which are a measure of muscle tension, are directly related to other physiological measures of autonomic arousal. It would be expected, therefore, that EMG levels of insomniacs would be greater than that of non-insomniacs. Insomnia may be associated with inadequate stimulus control of sleeping behaviors. That is, insomniacs may engage in a large number of behaviors incompatible with sleeping (e.g., eating, watching TV, reading) while in their bed and bedroom. The stimuli (i.e., bed and sleeping room) may become associated with these incompatible behaviors, thereby decreasing the probability

that the behavior of "going to sleep" will be emitted in those situations. The treatment of insomnia has historically been medically oriented (i.e., administration of tranquilizers or sedatives).

But here is the good news for insomniacs and non-insomniacs alike. Their paper also states:

Recently, however, several investigators have reported successful treatment of insomnia in a number of uncontrolled case studies using variants of systematic desensitization or relaxation training. The use of these behavioral techniques in the treatment of insomnia is based on the premise that anxiety or heightened autonomic arousal is an etiological or maintaining factor.

In other words, what we learn from reading the above few paragraphs is that everyone can sleep better with better self-care and personal attention to their sleep hygiene, and that learning how to relax is key to better sleep! Learning how to lower stress in our daily lives helps us to sleep better, as does learning how to control anxiety, fears, and worries.

The National Alliance on Mental Illness (NAMI) says:

One of the major sleep disorders that people face is insomnia. Insomnia is an inability to get the amount of sleep needed to function efficiently during the daytime. Insomnia is caused by difficulty falling asleep, difficulty staying asleep or waking up too early in the morning. Insomnia is rarely an isolated medical or mental illness but rather a symptom of another illness to be investigated by a person and their medical doctors. In other people, insomnia can be a result of a person's lifestyle or work schedule. Sometimes insomnia or other sleep problems can be caused by sleep apnea, which is a separate medical condition that affects a person's ability to breathe while sleeping. A doctor or sleep specialist can diagnose sleep apnea and provide treatment to improve sleep.

The National Sleep Foundation says: "About 1 in 3 people in the United States report difficulty sleeping at least one night per week, according to a recent study." You can explore this further, after a few nights' sleep, at www.sleepfoundation.org. As their site states, "The 2015 Sleep in America™ poll finds that pain joins two related concerns — stress and poor health — as key correlates of shorter sleep durations and worse sleep quality. But there are paths to resolving the problem: The sleep gap narrows sharply among those who *make sleep a priority*." You may also check out www.sleep.org, the foundation's new site.

The good news? You are still reading, and that definitely puts you in the group that "make sleep a priority." Hmm... are you hearing a lullaby yet?

Short-term insomnia is very common and has many causes such as stress, travel, or other sleep-disrupting life events. It can generally be relieved by simple sleep hygiene interventions such as exercise, a hot bath, warm milk, or changing your bedroom environment. Long-term insomnia lasts for more than three weeks and should be investigated by a physician with a potential referral to a sleep disorder specialist, which includes psychiatrists, neurologists, and pulmonologists who have expertise in sleep disorders.

We can't ignore hormonal issues preventing sleep, either. According to *Women's Health* magazine:

> Women may be more likely to have insomnia than men because women experience unique hormonal changes that can cause insomnia symptoms. These include hormonal changes during the menstrual cycle, especially in the days leading up to their period when many women report problems going to sleep and staying asleep.

While awareness of hormonal issues is indeed important, it is beyond the scope of this book to address them any further. There may be various medical solutions, and a sleep doctor may recommend specific remedies. Still, I urge you to first try conditioning your mind using the techniques presented in this book. The I Am Sleeping Now method works!

And what about sleep and pain? If you're asking this, great question! With clearance from your doctor or pain specialist, hypnosis is an evidence-based, widely proven modality for the treatment of chronic pain. Though not the subject of this book specifically, should you be experiencing chronic pain that impacts your ability to sleep, please consider the services of a professional hypnotist experienced in working in this area. I invite you to reach out so that we can explore how I may help you in reducing or eliminating chronic pain so you can both sleep better and enjoy your waking hours more! Best to send an email or call the office. I work with people directly in the office, and via video sessions over the internet as well.

Perhaps you are realizing, as you read, that it's time to break the grip of sleeplessness, chronic pain, and chronic insomnia. The health benefits of a good night's sleep are profound, and the health risks of failing to master sleep are troubling. Let's drop all invalid diagnoses, and let's apply hypnosis as a tool to help alleviate and eliminate chronic pain.

So, Let's Begin by Getting a Solid Baseline on Your Sleep

Examine these questions, at least briefly, because each one is important in helping you sleep better each night. Please be honest with yourself. Journey within and really try to answer each question. Your answers will help you achieve your sleep goals! Feel free to grab a pen, and then go ahead and write your answers either right here in the book or on a separate piece of paper. Answer each one!

1. What are your current sleeping habits and patterns?

2. How much sleep are you getting now?

3. When do you go to bed?

4. Are you on the internet or in social media groups seeking support or to self-diagnose and/or get sympathy for your sleeplessness? (Stop it!)

5. Do you set an alarm?

6. Are you generally a happy person?

7. Are you depressed or sad? Diagnosed with depression?

8. When did sleeping problems begin for you?

9. What does your pre-sleep routine look like?

10. What is keeping you from sleeping? (Your subconscious mind knows!)

11. Is your primary issue getting to sleep or staying asleep?

12. What could you change in your daily routines and habits that might help?

13. What are you afraid of, or worry about?

14. Are you sabotaging yourself with negative self-talk?

15. Are there any regrets, feelings and emotions, or forgiveness work to examine?

16. Are you considerably overweight? Overeating?

17. What about bad habits? What needs to change?

18. Is alcohol a problem?

19. Do you go to bed at the same time each night?

20. Seriously, what needs to be addressed in your life so you can sleep better?

21. Are there any other habits that are preventing you from enjoying a good night's sleep?

22. I wonder whether you believe yet that you can train your mind and body to sleep?

23. Is there something that needs to be addressed in your life so you can sleep better?

In the quiet moments I want you to listen to your heart, your mind, and your body. Listen to your spiritual side as well. Settle into the silence to hear the conversation your subconscious mind is wanting to have with you. You see, with congruence, alignment, and clarity of intention, your mind will help you become physically and mentally relaxed, inviting sleep to your abode.

As a professional hypnotist, I help people resolve all kinds of issues in large part by helping them improve the communication with their own subconscious mind. You see, on a deep subconscious level, there is a part of you that knows (or has a very good hunch) what is preventing you from entering the realm of sleep. No worries, though! I AM SLEEPING NOW will help you relax and set aside anything on your mind.

Here are some more important questions that will help you resolve or let go of whatever it may be that is keeping you from sleep:

- When did your sleep struggle first begin? Recently, or weeks, months, or years ago?
- What was going on in your life at that time?
- Are there unresolved issues, or feelings that deserve re-examination?
- What feelings are you aware of as your day ends and sleep-time is just ahead?

Trust the process. Trust the suggestions in this book, keep reading, and practice, practice, practice. Sleep awaits you!

CHAPTER TWO

Let Aesop Lull You Into Your Sleep Mindset

"Like those who dine well of the plainest dishes, Aesop made use of humble incidents to teach great truths; by announcing a story which everyone knows not to be true, he told the truth by the very fact that he did not claim to be relating real events."
—Philostratus, *Life of Apollonius of Tyana*, Book V:14

A good night's sleep sets us up for a better tomorrow, allowing us to awaken recharged, rejuvenated, and reenergized, with greater resilience. And a good power nap improves the next phase of our day or evening. Executives and businesses, along with people from various walks of life, know the importance and the secrets of grabbing a nod when they need one. It's good common-sense wisdom that is, well, not too common, unfortunately, when you consider the sleeplessness that surrounds us.

Aesop knew this and shared his fables to pass along the wisdom of revering sleep.

As Philostratus said centuries ago, stories well told are great teachers. Aesop, a great teacher himself, told oral stories that were designed to make a strong impact. Good stories and metaphors set us up for hearing messages and meanings, subconsciously, in a way that our conscious mind struggles to embrace. Thus, storytelling throughout the ages has been a powerful tool in passing down generational wisdom, morals, and values, and even lull us to invite and embrace sleep so easily. (By the way, I wonder what stories you are telling yourself which may, in fact, be *preventing* you from enjoying a good night's sleep?)

As a professional hypnotist, I frequently tell various types of stories to my clients as a therapeutic tool in the change work we do together. I share relevant client stories to convey that others have faced challenges similar to their own, for instance, and whether I'm working with children or adults, I have also found that one very powerful storytelling tool as well is the fable, and specifically Aesop's Fables. You recall Aesop, right? Remember some of his fables?

Aesop's Fables, if you are new to Aesop, are short, high-impact stories rich in allegory featuring mostly animals as main characters in place of humans. Giving non-human characters voice and applying to them person-like traits in this way (called anthropomorphization) is a clever and useful storytelling device. It has the wonderful effect of lowering the human reader's resistance to any underlying message the tale may have, and thus the mind becomes more accepting of the story's meaning for possible future relevance and applicability. Make sense?

Aesop (620–564 B.C.) is legendary, and while his fables were never originally meant for children, through the ages they have been recast as children's stories. Perhaps you have read his fables to your children or have been on the receiving end of a fable or two as a child.

The magic of Aesop's Fables lies in their easy-to-understand morals, which the listener hears and applies as the mind sees fit. Some of the more familiar fables, as you may recall, include:

- "The Ant and the Grasshopper"
- "The Boy Who Cried Wolf"
- "The Fox and the Crow"
- "The Fox and the Grapes"
- "The Honest Woodcutter"
- "The North Wind and the Sun"
- "The Tortoise and the Hare"
- "The Town Mouse and the Country Mouse"

It becomes clear that Aesop was focused on the importance of sleep some 2,500 years ago, as we see this theme reflected in at least several of his fables, along with the morals or lessons to be found therein. While it is true that his fables have been rewritten and re-imagined over the span of time to become children's stories, they have universal appeal and apply to all. So be careful not to dismiss his works, as the stories just might help you sleep! Aesop's fables address the human struggles of sleep, and his lessons may very well transform your life in this area and others, as my aptly-titled book, *The Magic of Aesop: How to Use the Wisdom of Aesop's Fables to Spark Your Transformational Change*, so ably suggests. (Get *The Magic of Aesop* at Amazon or at bobmartel.com.)

Before exploring a small handful of Aesop's Fables, consider this great spin on one of them: A major furniture store recently launched a campaign across the UK to promote the benefits of sleep. Of course, their main goal was in selling more mattresses, bed frames, and other such bedroom items. But the brilliant ad campaign in question is worth noting here because it creatively hacked my favorite Aesop's Fable, "The Tortoise and the Hare."

Let me begin by sharing that particular fable from Aesop for both your enjoyment and edification.

The Tortoise and the Hare

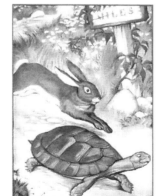

Milo Winter (1919)

A Hare one day ridiculed the short feet and slow pace of the Tortoise. The latter, laughing, said: "Though you be swift as the wind, I will beat you in a race." The Hare, deeming her

35

assertion to be simply impossible, assented to the proposal; and they agreed that the Fox should choose the course and fix the goal. On the day appointed for the race they started together. The Tortoise never for a moment stopped but went on with a slow but steady pace straight to the end of the course. The Hare, trusting to his native swiftness, cared little about the race, and lying down by the wayside, fell fast asleep. At last waking up, and moving as fast as he could, he saw the Tortoise had reached the goal, and was comfortably dozing *after* her fatigue.

Let me present another version:

A Hare was making fun of the Tortoise one day for being so slow.

"Do you ever get anywhere?" he asked with a mocking laugh.

"Yes," replied the Tortoise, "and I get there sooner than you think. I'll run you a race and prove it."

The Hare was much amused at the idea of running a race with the Tortoise, but for the fun of the thing he agreed. So, the Fox, who had consented to act as judge, marked the distance and started the runners off.

The Hare was soon far out of sight, and to make the Tortoise feel very deeply how ridiculous it was for him to try a race with a Hare, he lay down beside the course to take a nap until the Tortoise should catch up.

The Tortoise meanwhile kept going slowly but steadily, and, after a time, passed the place *where the Hare was sleeping*. But the Hare slept on very peacefully; and when at last, he did wake up, the Tortoise was near the goal. The Hare now ran his swiftest, but he could not overtake the Tortoise in time.

Moral of the story: The race is not always to the swift.

Re-read the above two versions of Aesop's fable quickly. Notice the word *sleep*. Now, notice how this might be relevant in your life, or not.

Now back to the Tortoise and the Hare 'hack' by the British advertising agency in its campaign for IKEA furniture. There's a great new moral featured in the ad's modern twist on this famous fable, and that moral is: "Tomorrow Starts Tonight."

(Yes, your tomorrow starts tonight! So keep reading, and let's get you sleeping better!)

The imaginative and creative marketing team takes you to the night *prior to* the celebrated Hare and Tortoise race. Their prequel to the great race illustrates an important lesson or decision point for anyone facing an important day ahead. In fact, it's a great story about respecting and revering sleep as an important part of our waking life. The Tortoise turns in for a good night's sleep, anticipating the next day's race. The next morning, he is calm, relaxed, confident, and ready for the big day. He leaves the house with running gear, and a racing number on his jersey. He's ready! The Hare, on the other hand, stays out partying late, playing video games into the night, fighting off the desire to sleep, convinced he'll easily win the race!

As the ad agency's marketing communication manager says, in an IKEA story about the video, "Stress and anxiety can have a really damaging effect on sleep, which in turn impacts our waking life too. A good night's sleep sets us up for a great next day, and the new integrated campaign aims to help people find ways to prioritize sleep. There really is a lot of truth in the notion that a brilliant day starts the night before."

Find the 1:32-minute video for the ad online, if you'd like, by searching "Ikea video furniture ad The Hare."

"The Tortoise and the Hare" is one of Aesop's most famous and most fabulous fables and is numbered 226 in the Perry Index (explained in my book, *The Magic of Aesop*). The fable itself is a variant of a common folktale theme in which ingenuity and/or trickery are employed to overcome a stronger opponent. While the account of a race between unequal partners has attracted conflicting interpretations through the ages, most focus on the dangers of foolish overconfidence (as illustrated by the Hare) and the virtues of perseverance (as nobly demonstrated by the Tortoise).

Hmmm. I wonder how better sleep can help you overcome adversaries, real and imagined, past, present, and future?

I wonder, too, and am curious about whether you turn in consistently for a decent night's sleep in order to prepare yourself for that next big day ahead. A good night's sleep is essential to a better day. *Tomorrow starts tonight.*

The Fox and the Grapes

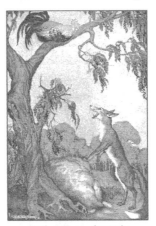

Milo Winter (1919)

A Fox one day spied a beautiful bunch of ripe grapes hanging from a vine trained along the branches of a tree. The grapes seemed ready to burst with juice, and the Fox's mouth watered as he gazed longingly at them.

The bunch hung from a high branch, and the Fox had to jump for it. The first time he jumped he missed it by a long way. So he walked off a short distance and took a running leap at it, only to fall short once more. Again and again he tried, but in vain.

Now he sat down and looked at the grapes in disgust.

"What a fool I am," he said. "Here I am wearing myself out to get a bunch of sour grapes that are not worth gaping for."

And off he walked very, very scornfully.

Moral: It is easy to despise what you believe you cannot get.

The Fox was going for low-hanging fruit and rather than work for the real prize, instead rationalized his 'truth' and simply surmised the grapes were not worth the effort!

When it comes to your pursuit of falling and staying asleep using the power of your mind to do so, you must acknowledge that you will make the effort, because the results are so worth it!

The North Wind and the Sun

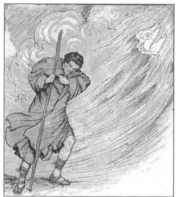

Milo Winter (1919)

A dispute once arose between the North Wind and the Sun as to which was the stronger of the two. Seeing a traveler on his way, they agreed to try which could the sooner get his cloak off him. The North Wind began, and sent a furious blast, which, at the onset, nearly tore the cloak from its fastenings; but the traveler, seizing the garment with a firm grip, held it round his body so tightly that Boreas spent his remaining force in vain. The Sun, dispelling the clouds that had gathered, then darted his most sultry beams on the traveler's head. Growing faint with the heat, the man flung off his cloak, and ran for protection to the nearest shade.

Moral: Sometimes gentle persuasion might work better than the strongest force.

As you continue your journey of learning to sleep like a baby once again, I wonder if this Aesop's Fable offers a message for your resourceful subconscious mind. Hmmm.

The Owl and the Grasshopper

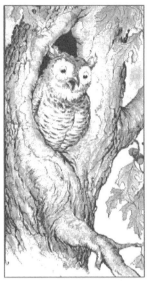

Milo Winter (1919)

The Owl always takes her sleep during the day. Then after sundown, when the rosy light fades from the sky and the shadows rise slowly through the wood, out she comes ruffling and blinking from the old hollow tree. Now her weird "hoo-hoo-hoo-oo-oo" echoes through the quiet wood, and she begins her hunt for the bugs and beetles, frogs and mice she likes so well to eat.

Now there was a certain old Owl who had become very cross and hard to please as she grew older, especially if anything disturbed her daily slumbers. One warm summer afternoon as she dozed away in her den in the old oak tree, a Grasshopper nearby began a joyous but very raspy song. Out popped the old Owl's head from the opening in the tree that served her both for door and for window.

"Get away from here, sir," she said to the Grasshopper. "Have you no manners? You should at least respect my age and leave me to sleep in quiet!"

But the Grasshopper answered saucily that he had as much right to his place in the sun as the Owl had to her

40

place in the old oak. Then he struck up a louder and still more rasping tune.

The wise old Owl knew quite well that it would do no good to argue with the Grasshopper, nor with anybody else for that matter. Besides, her eyes were not sharp enough by day to permit her to punish the Grasshopper as he deserved. So she laid aside all hard words and spoke very kindly to him.

"Well, sir," she said, "if I must stay awake, I am going to settle right down to enjoy your singing. Now that I think of it, I have a wonderful wine here, sent me from Olympus, of which I am told Apollo drinks before he sings to the high gods. Please come up and taste this delicious drink with me. I know it will make you sing like Apollo himself."

The foolish Grasshopper was taken in by the Owl's flattering words. Up he jumped to the Owl's den, but as soon as he was near enough so the old Owl could see him clearly, she pounced upon him and ate him up. Then the Owl finished her nap in comfort.

Moral: While it appears to be a violent ending for the Grasshopper, the Owl solved the problem by addressing the problem head-on!

In the still of your own quiet moments, I wonder if this Aesop's Fable has any special meaning? Are there metaphorical Grasshoppers that need to be addressed in your waking hours so they do not continue to pester you when sleep time arrives?

I suggest you consider this fable a way for you to accept the "Grasshopper" as those things that prevent you from quieting your mind. Trust my process as you read, confident that you will learn to achieve sleep mastery by calming your mind and body, and achieve it rather quickly, I might add!

And that's just a short introduction to the value of Aesop's Fables. Explore his great works after you've completed the Seven-Day Challenge, or at some point down the road. Of course, I recommend you start with *The Magic of Aesop*!

And while I do not expect you to recite fables to yourself as you fall asleep, you certainly can get lost in a story you weave, as a tool or strategy for clearing your mind as you invite sleep to your pillow. Our mind enjoys a good story. It occupies our attention, which is the very point, and then allows, in this case, for our body to fall asleep naturally.

Here's an example...

Zzz-Tip: Occasionally, I will use a mind-occupying story to ease myself into sleep. Imagine this. I'll get physically comfortable, take a few comforting breaths, and close my eyes. I'll imagine or retrace all the places I have traveled to by airplane, in chronological order, to the best of my recollection, and without letting my mind ruminate on any of the details at any given destination. Let me restate the steps:

- Breathe to relax.
- Get physically comfortable.
- Focus on mental relaxation.
- Occupy the mind with a simple "drill," or mental field trip.

In my own mental field trip, while inviting sleep to my pillow, I experience my head hitting the pillow as an anchor to put me in the sleep mode. Spinning a distracting story, I always start out in Boston and travel to Orlando, to Navy bootcamp at seventeen, and then back to Boston. Then to San Diego for training, home again and back to San Diego, up to San Francisco for more training, and to Groton, Connecticut for submarine school. If I am not already asleep by then (I usually fade before getting to Groton), I will then retrace additional flying destinations from later in my life. Boston to San Francisco to catch a flight to Tokyo, Singapore, Seoul, Hong Kong, Sydney, or to London, Munich, Stockholm, Milan, Belfast, or Geneva. I seldom get this far, but it's nice to have a story to continue if the first few stops don't do the trick.

You get the idea. You'll develop your own mental field trip to occupy your mind as sleep comes a-knockin'. Recall or create a journey you can take in your mind, a mental field trip, so to speak. Something light and positive. The trick is simply to focus your mind's attention while your intention to fall asleep becomes real.

We will be building on this theme of mental conditioning and mind–body training to help you sleep better.

Hopefully, you have enjoyed this chapter. The point is this:

- What calming stories can you use to quiet your mind as you begin to go to sleep?
- What sleep-preventing stories are you allowing to fester in your mind?
- What stories are you entertaining in your waking life that are the cause of angst, anxiety, stress, and general unhappiness?

CHAPTER THREE

Your Journey to Saqqara – Imhotep Was Right!

"Never go to sleep without a request to your subconscious."
—Thomas Edison, 1847–1931, American inventor

Your subconscious mind is always alert, and when your intention is *"SLEEP,"* it stands ready to help make that happen! The ancient healers discovered this in their sleep temples!

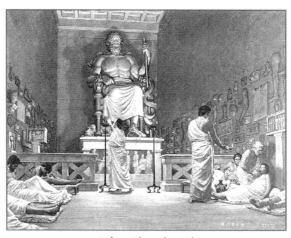

Robert Thom (1957)

In fact, long before Thomas Edison shared the observation quoted above, people in ancient civilizations realized this same wisdom. Since the beginning of mankind, in whatever words or images they used at the time, it was well known that quieting the mind was crucial to falling and staying asleep. There was an embracing of a positive attitude and a reverence for the ritual of preparing for sleep.

It's still true today!

Here's the magic.

The whole secret to my time-tested and well-proven method is based on Edison's general observation, in that too many people who struggle with sleep (most, in fact) fail to enlist the help of the subconscious mind. They chase sleep consciously, instead of inviting it into their realm subconsciously as they should. The mind and body work closely together, as we well know, and the power of our very intention to fall asleep is a signal to the subconscious. Consider it a request for help! When you follow your new pre-sleep process — as you will tailor, using the instructions throughout this book as your guide — you will condition yourself to drift into slumberland easily and effortlessly.

You might be wondering why this book needs a section on a historical discussion of sleep via the words and wisdom of such preeminent figures as Edison. And who is this fellow Imhotep, anyway, as mentioned in the chapter title? And where is Saqqara, for that matter, and why would we wish to journey there? Why is any of this even relevant?

Stay with me, please!

I ask that you *trust the process*, please, as you continue your journey toward sleep mastery. Suggestion therapy, or what is also referred to as hypnosis, goes back much further than the days of Franz Anton Mesmer, who was considered the father of hypnosis by some. Self-suggestions, which are an integral part of your sleep mastery, will be taught as we go. Mankind has been pursuing the benefits of the sleep state since the beginning, and the ancient Egyptians and Greeks documented their healing success using sleep as their tool for success. You are on your way to doing the same!

It's important to acknowledge that even ancient civilizations struggled with sleeplessness, which is my point in this chapter. Believe it or not, you are connected to the intentions of those who came before you, all of whom were also seeking the same thing!

You share a commonality with billions of people throughout the ages who sought the peace and harmony of restful, healing sleep. Utilizing the trance state to help access the powerful benefits of sleep goes back thousands of years — a bit of a mystery then, and in some ways still a mystery today. Even in Greek mythology it was acknowledged that Hypnos, the primordial god of sleep, was to be revered. Your sleep deserves nothing less.

It was the Egyptian physician and architect Imhotep who led the Sleep Temple or Dream Temple movement back in the days of the pharaoh Djoser, the first king of the Third Dynasty, circa 2670 B.C. Imhotep's sleep temples were among early medicine's healing modalities. Even the king's staff wrote of sleep! A hieroglyphic inscription down the center of an ancient papyrus reads: "Good Sleeping in the West, the Land of Righteousness," by the Royal Scribe Qenherkhepeshef.

In ancient times, the temple sleep was used as a psychotherapeutic tool, and the temples of Imhotep were well attended by people looking for psychological help. Under the influence of incantation and the performance of religious rituals, sick people were prepared psychologically for suggestion therapy by being put into what we'd now call a hypnotic state. Before falling asleep, they were influenced by suggestions in the hopes of provoking dreams sent by the gods.

Imagine if Imhotep and his fellow priests had access to this book then! The phrase "I am sleeping now" would have worked like magic for his subjects then, as it is helping you now! I am sure they had their own magical hypnotic suggestions and rituals!

It is said that once Djoser took the throne, he needed a builder, and Imhotep was his man. This Egyptian high priest became a busy guy with grand plans to develop the region. Historian Margaret Bunson writes that Djoser "ruled during an age witnessing advances in civilization on the Nile such as the construction of architectural monuments, agricultural developments, trade, and the rise of the cities." It was Djoser who commissioned Imhotep to build the Step Pyramid complex of Saqqara, where the sleep temples were located.

Imhotep, and his fellow priests and priestesses, used sleep to heal the whole person. They called it incubation, or temple sleep — sleeping in a sacred space to access healing through the dream appearance of the healer. It was considered a consultation of the oracles, where the answers to their healing were received in a dream.

This wasn't something unique to the Egyptians, either. Later on, for instance, in this practice known as temple sleep, ailing people came to dream in oracular temples such as those devoted to the Greek god of medicine, Asclepius. There, they performed rites or sacrifices in efforts to dream appropriately, and they then slept in wait of the appearance of the god (or his emissary). They lay down to sleep in the dormitory, or *abaton*, and were visited in their dreams by Asclepius or by one of his priests, who gave advice. In the morning, the patient was often said to have departed the temple cured. Of course, we know now that this trance state we call hypnosis is a tool for helping the conscious and subconscious mind to align, communicate, and achieve congruence, all to make progress toward your goal.

How does this pertain to you?

Well, in our case, the goal is to fall and stay asleep! And here, in this modern age, we can utilize these same tools of hypnosis toward that end. I want you to start picturing sleep success in your mind. How will you feel awakening after a good night's sleep? Know that this good feeling *is going to happen*. Visualize it. Connect with it. Bring those future feelings to today.

I'll let you further explore Asclepius and Imhotep and Saqqara on your own. This book, and your effort to find that elusive sleep, is your journey to Saqqara. It is merely a metaphor; you are going to Saqqara in your mind.

You see, if Franz Mesmer (from whence the term "mesmerized" is derived) can be called the father of hypnosis, then the great, great, great grandfather of hypnosis could arguably be considered the ancient Egyptian priest Imhotep. Imhotep, whose name means "the one who comes in peace," gets credit for discovering the benefits of early hypnotic healing in the sleep temples he built for King Djoser.

What does all of this have to do with you getting a good night's sleep?

It is this: Imagine your bedroom as a sleep temple, your sacred place to repair, rejuvenate, heal, and reenergize so you can greet the day tomorrow refreshed. Just as the Greek and Egyptian priests and priestesses of long ago used healing sanctuaries to help people resolve all sorts of physical and mental issues, I wonder if you can also look at your sleep state with the same type of reverence and importance that it deserves. (I say this because so many of the clients I help with sleep issues complain about sleeplessness yet continue to sabotage their own sleep success.) What say you?

Sometimes our current subconscious behavior prevents us from making progress toward our conscious intentions. It is then that we must *de*-hypnotize ourselves from old, unwanted patterns, and then take back control by using hypnotic techniques to give our mind new, *better* suggestions that are much more in alignment with what we want for ourselves.

The key is to focus on what we *want*, and not on what we do *not* want. We get more of what we focus upon — meaning it is better to visualize and connect with how it will feel, each day better and better, as you begin to enjoy waking from a good night's sleep. *Where the attention goes, the energy flows.* Always remember that!

What's Old Is New Again: Hypnosis Still Works!

One could argue that Imhotep and his band of high priests used what we today call hypnosis, and the power of therapeutic sleep to help people to heal. In many ways, sleep is as mysterious now as it was at the time of the Step Pyramids and sleep temples. Hypnosis, however, is now an evidence-based, well-proven tool for change work!

Hypnosis, as I hope you'll be open to accepting, is the key to falling and staying asleep, and to reconditioning your mind and body to be calm, relaxed, and harmoniously at peace within when you invite sleep to your pillow.

Hypnosis is, at its core, a heightened state of awareness and focused concentration, which allows the mind to consider and embrace new suggestions, all in the context of the client's highest and best, and with their conscious intention at the forefront. The subconscious mind processes feelings and emotions, it stores our automatic habitual patterns and programs, and it serves to protect us.

In this book, although not a comprehensive tutorial on the use of hypnosis as a whole, you will learn enough to master the skills of physical and mental relation, of calming the mind, and of programming yourself to sleep when the time for sleep arrives. We'll talk more about helpful self-hypnosis techniques in this regard in subsequent chapters.

As you might already be aware, the phrase "I am sleeping now" is a powerful, positive, present-tense example of a hypnotic suggestion you can use to make that statement become your reality as your head hits the pillow. File that idea for now. We'll get to it shortly.

"*I am sleeping now*" will become an automatic auditory anchor, whether you say it silently or aloud, and will certainly become such as you recite this phrase to yourself repeatedly. You will see this as you journey to your sleep temple. It is a positive, present-tense affirmation.

Imagine this for now. In the days of Imhotep, the people entering the sleep temple walked a beautiful path designed to relax them, and to focus them on the experience that lay ahead. They had anticipation, great hope, and an expectation.

Zzz-Tip: It's time for you to see your journey to your bedroom as an anchor that focuses you on what comes next — a good night's sleep. Make it a positive, self-fulfilling prophecy. Enter your sleep domain knowing that every day, and in every way, you are getting better and better at sleeping soundly. All negative thoughts and all negative self-talk fade, for you are conditioning your mind and body, through nightly practice, to easily fall and stay asleep.

Imagine, also, those people entering the sleep temples long ago. They prepared for their experience. You can (and must) do the same. For now, let's call it your pre-sleep routine and rituals — those things you add or subtract from your evening activities to prepare yourself for sleep.

Start to embrace the idea of adopting wise pre-sleep habits, and your habits and behaviors of the day. Perhaps starting your waking state when you arise from sleep with a positive intention that will drive your purpose for the whole day. For example, what if you said to yourself each morning: "Every day and in every way, I am better and better."

> *"Fatigue is the best pillow."*
> —Benjamin Franklin

Benjamin Franklin was a master of productivity and followed a rigid schedule, including his sleep time. He slept from 10:00 p.m. to 5:00 a.m. each night, according to his memoirs. In the morning he asked himself, "What good shall I do this day?" And he ended the day by asking himself, "What good have I done today?" Two great questions to consider for peace of mind each evening as you hit the pillow!

Here are a handful of quotes from some other great thinkers whose perception of sleep may positively influence you:

> "Man should forget his anger before he lies down to sleep."
> —Mahatma Gandhi

> "Many things — such as loving, going to sleep, or behaving unaffectedly — are done worst when we try hardest to do them."
> —C. S. Lewis

> "If you can't sleep, then get up and do something instead of lying there worrying. It's the worry that gets you, not the lack of sleep."
> —Dale Carnegie

"Don't fight with the pillow, but lay down your head. And kick every worriment out of the bed."
—Edmund Vance Cooke

"A dying man needs to die, as a sleepy man needs to sleep, and there comes a time when it is wrong, as well as useless, to resist."
—Stewart Alsop

"When I want to go to sleep, I must first get a whole menagerie of voices to shut up. You wouldn't believe what a racket they make in my room."
—Karl Kraus

"Sleep is the best meditation."
—Dalai Lama

"The worst thing in the world is to try to sleep and not to."
—F. Scott Fitzgerald

"O sleep, O gentle sleep,
Nature's soft nurse, how have I frighted thee,
That thou no more wilt weigh my eyelids down
And steep my sense in forgetfulness?"
—William Shakespeare, *Henry IV, Part I*

Sage advice lies above. Agree? Long before Yoda said there was no trying, only doing, F. Scott Fitzgerald expressed a somewhat similar sentiment.

Stop trying to go to sleep and just go to sleep. Be open to shifting your perception of sleep as you continue reading.

Zzz-TIP: I realize that not everyone has the same attitude about the importance of sleep. Insomnia is an age-old problem. But apart from a diagnosis of any physical issues preventing slumber, you are indeed ready to begin the process of programming yourself to sleep better. A key part of this process in bringing quality sleep back into your life — without the need for dangerous side effect-laden sleep medication — lies in how you embrace the very notion of sleep:

- Is your self-talk aligned with your intention to sleep better again?
- Are you negatively programming yourself to be a chronic insomniac by the very words you use when the inner discussion turns to the topic of sleep?
- Are you sabotaging yourself in any way?

CHAPTER FOUR

Fall Asleep Fast: The U.S. Military Finds a Sleep Solution

"We sleep soundly in our beds because rough men stand ready in the night to visit violence on those who would do us harm."
—Sir Winston Churchill

Although often attributed to Churchill, it may not be his actual words above but, nonetheless, it speaks to the value and importance of safe and secure sleep. Ultimately, those guarding those asleep need their sleep as well. Everyone needs good sleep, to function well during the waking hours. (You know that!)

Let's get right to the point of this book now and focus on the sleeping technique that will have you off to dreamland within two minutes, once you've mastered it.

It's amazingly simple.

While you may or may not be active-duty military, there is a strong and relevant parallel here. You see, military personnel and civilians both need sleep! You may not be on a military mission, but you are on a mission called life, and if you want to maximize the quality of your daily living, what the military knows and embraces culturally applies to you as well. Science is science, and best practices apply universally.

If the U.S. military can teach the troops how to fall asleep fast, you should be able to use their time-tested methods too! The technique is easy to learn but mastery takes time, patience, and practice. Remember, the technique you are about to learn took an average of six weeks for skills mastery. You will learn it in seven days when you follow my guidance later in this book!

Imagine you being able to fall asleep at the drop of a hat, as the old expression goes, anywhere you find yourself. Mastering the technique in this chapter will require investment and commitment, but it will yield tremendous benefits throughout your life.

During the early days of America's involvement in World War II, in the European theatre, sleep-deprived fighter pilots were apparently shooting down friendly airplanes. The lack of sleep was causing poor performance, bad judgment, and allied planes were sent spiraling to the ground. Thus, grabbing some quality shut-eye became a priority. It was a matter of life and death.

The military brought in a naval officer, Lloyd C. "Bud" Winter, to teach relaxation techniques to Navy pilots. He was regarded as an expert in teaching people to stay calm under pressure, to think better, to feel better, and to win. Just the right thing for the squadrons trying to win the peace back then! (In his post-war career, Winter authored the famous book *Relax and Win: Championship Performance in Whatever You Do*, with co-author Jimson Lee.) Winter's method worked well for 96 percent of the pilots who practiced it for six weeks.

Of course, sleeping in a bed is always best, but it's not always an option. This simple relaxation technique, which really describes a brief self-hypnosis session on the pillow (if one is available), can be used sitting on a chair, on a plane, on a train, in your favorite recliner, or maybe even on a nice comfy blanket at the beach.

Here are the "fall asleep fast" relaxation steps comparable to what Bud Winter taught to U.S. military personnel. Before you begin this process, take a couple of nice relaxing breaths.

And now:

1. Get comfortable in your bed, and then relax all the muscles in your face. Feel all 43 of your facial muscles begin to relax deeply. Your brain will sense this relaxation.
   a. Choose your favorite sleeping position, if the situation allows.

    b. Sleeping on your back is best for this, but this is not essential.

    c. Most importantly, begin to focus on rapid physical relaxation.

    d. Let your chin and jaw become loose and relaxed.

2. Drop your shoulders and let them rest to continue the process.

    a. Feel yourself sinking deeper into the bed as you relax a little more.

    b. Focus on letting all muscle tension begin to dissipate and dissolve.

    c. Allow your arms, hands, and the muscles in your neck to begin to relax more deeply. You may even want to gently clench and unclench your hands and toes as you do this, unclenching as you release the tension while you focus on that tension leaving you. It's a nice feeling to enjoy.

3. Breathe.

    a. A full belly breath or two to continue the process will jumpstart the relaxation response as your body senses your intention to relax and drift toward sleep.

4. Relax your legs and feet deeply.

    a. Let your whole body relax as you feel your thighs, knees, calves, and feet relax, all the way down to your toes.

5. Clear your mind for 10–60 seconds.

    a. Be still physically while you focus on relaxing mentally.

    b. Ah! The hard part! You can train your brain to control your thoughts by focusing on other thoughts.

    c. Bud Winter had specific recommendations for clearing the mind:

       "First, we want you to fantasize that it is a warm spring day and you are lying in the bottom of a canoe on a very serene lake. You are looking up at a blue sky with lazy, floating clouds. Do not allow any other thought to creep in. Just concentrate on this picture and keep foreign thoughts out, particularly thoughts with any movement or motion involved. Hold this picture and enjoy it for 10 seconds.

"In the second sleep-producing fantasy, imagine that you are in a big, black, velvet hammock and everywhere you look is black. You must also hold this picture for 10 seconds.

"The third trick is to say the words *'don't think... don't think... don't think,'* etc. Hold this, blanking out other thoughts for at least 10 seconds."

Seems simple. It *is* amazingly simple! We will be using self-hypnosis plus the above method to help you take back control and sleep on command!

There is much to discuss regarding each of these five steps outlined above, and we will do so — later. (Later in Chapter Ten, for instance, you'll discover more self-hypnotic techniques to add to the military's fast sleeping drill. Stay with me for now and trust the process!)

Winter's technique is, essentially, an abbreviated progressive muscle relaxation technique commonly used to start the relaxation response, jumpstarting the calming of the mind and body. This will be explored on a deeper level in a later chapter as well.

In the modern era, business leaders have discovered the benefits of a good night's sleep for their employees. While certainly not a new concept in general, they kept this secret and applied it only to themselves for centuries, always making sure *they* got enough sleep, but being little concerned about their labor force. It's only within the last 20 years or so that executives and business owners have decided to focus on the sleep quality of not just themselves, but of their employees as well. After all, it makes sense!

- Accidents are reduced.
- Absenteeism is lowered.
- Morale is up, and complaints are down.
- Profits are up. Those who run corporate America want you to get a good night's sleep, but for their benefit, not yours, no matter how they sugarcoat it. Google "executive sleep"

and enjoy the tangential adventure — *after* finishing your sleep mastery lessons here in this book.

Let's get back to what the military learned from their WWII sleep training. It is still a part of military training today. In fact, the U.S. Army, in their field manual *FM 7-22: Holistic Health and Fitness*, a publication available to everyone, focuses on sleep readiness as a strategic weapon on the battlefield. But it goes back, way before being implemented by the sleep experts during WWII. Sleep has always been a mission X-factor in the military, and just plain smart. Done right, it kept you ready, and alive!

As John "Gunner" Starnes writes in his documentation of the early history of the Airborne Rangers, "In 1759, a young but experienced Major Robert Rogers formed nine companies of rangers and 'for their benefit and instruction reduced into writing the following rules, or plans of discipline.' These standing orders were developed from Rogers' experiences during the French and Indian War, and he considered them 'necessary and advantageous.' Robert Rogers' standing orders for his Rangers are still valid today."

Rogers' 28 "Rules of Ranging" and his associated "Standing Orders" included several provisions about sleep! I mention this for one reason only — to further illustrate the importance of sleep, as viewed by professionals in the most dangerous of scenarios, the battlefield. If those who protect us can master their sleep skills, so can you — with the same discipline and commitment!

The courageous Robert Rogers, the founding father of today's special forces military approach, was a major influence on Merrill's Marauders in WWII, and prior to that, he influenced the Corps of Rangers formed by Daniel Morgan and his famous "crack shots" credited with helping to win the Battle of Saratoga.

I'll resist the temptation to say too much more about this particular subject, so as to keep on track on the topic of sleep! Certainly, it may be more than you need to know to help you sleep, but please bear with me. The history lesson is relevant in that among those early Ranger units — which included amidst their ranks such notables as Daniel Boone and Abraham Lincoln! — sleep was revered.

In 1776, Knowlton's Rangers of the Continental Army adopted many of Rogers' rules and tactics, and today's U.S. Army Rangers revere sleep and know how to grab some ZZZs when they are able. The topic of sleep has long been recognized as both strategic and life-saving for them. Same applies to you.

Rangers Lead the Way, as their motto says, and that includes getting proper sleep. While this book is not intended to make you think like an Army Ranger, there is a lot to be gained by adopting a similar mindset in regard to sleep. Straight from the Ranger Handbook (which, under the handbook's title, states: "Not for the weak or fainthearted") the Army addresses sleep as such:

- Rest/Sleep Plan Management. The patrol conducts rest as necessary to prepare for future operations.
  [In other words, sleep and naps are mission-critical. —Bob]

- With the will to survive, you will find you can overcome any obstacle you may face. You will survive. You must understand the emotional states associated with survival; "knowing thyself" is extremely important in a survival situation. It bears directly on how well you cope with serious stresses, anxiety, pain, injury, illness; cold, heat, thirst, hunger, fatigue, sleep deprivation, boredom, loneliness and isolation.

As the U.S. Army teaches its soldiers and leaders, taken directly from Chapter 11 of *FM 7-22: Holistic Health and Fitness*:

> The brain is the only organ or body part that requires sleep. Sleep is crucial for tissue repair and hormone synthesis to maintain peak performance mentally and physically. Sleep sustains brain and physical health, cognition, the immune system, and recovery after physical activity. This chapter provides tools and techniques for leaders and individuals exercising sleep readiness tactics, techniques, and procedures for a range of occupations and operational environments.

Sleep Readiness for Soldiers & Sailors Applies to *Everyone*

Sleep is considered a force multiplier by all branches of the military. It can be, and will soon become once again, your force multiplier as well, enabling you to accomplish amazing things. Military leaders are taught and reminded of the importance of sleep in regard to mission success. That same wisdom applies to you also. Revering sleep and getting enough of it are two key points I want you to embrace in this chapter.

Sleep is well studied by the military. If your area of interest extends beyond your personal sleep mastery goals and intentions and you wish to learn more, I recommend downloading and reading the U.S. Navy's *Sleep Management User's Guide for Special Operations Personnel*, first published in 1963 by the Naval Health Research Center, Special Operations Division. It is all still quite relevant today — for both military and civilian use! You can find the full report, filled with sage advice, by searching for the title.

Whether a soldier, sailor, airman, or Marine, sleep mastery is key. Like them, you need adequate sleep to maintain your own operational readiness and mission success. *Your* mission is to get enough sleep each night that your waking hours are happy and productive. It's all about resilience and being in the optimal wake state to perform or function well. Before going any further, why not add the words "reliance," "perseverance," "determination," and "tenacity" to your core principles?

More from FM 7-22:

> Soldiers should sleep as much as they can, whenever they can, as the situation allows. The vast majority of Soldiers require 7–8 hours of sleep per night to sustain performance; more sleep is better. Soldiers can maximize sleep and subsequent performance by timing sleep and caffeine use optimally. Finally, only sleep replaces lost sleep.

Self-care includes proper sleep. It's true for the military, as the U.S. Army and the U.S. Naval Institute note, and it is true for you as well. You are the captain of your own ship — your life! — and the captain of a naval ship is in command of both the mission and the ship. You are, indeed, the captain of your soul, as William Ernest Henley so eloquently shares in his most famous work, "Invictus," published in his first volume of poems, *Book of Verses*, and featured later on, amongst other notable entries, in *The Voice of Science in Nineteenth Century Literature*. Ah, I digress a bit as I write this chapter, I know, but you may enjoy Henley's words:

Invictus

Out of the night that covers me,
Black as a Pit from pole to pole,
I thank whatever gods may be
For my unconquerable soul.

In the fell clutch of circumstance
I have not winced nor cried aloud.
Under the bludgeonings of chance
My head is bloody, but unbowed.

Beyond this place of wrath and tears
Looms but the Horror of the shade,
And yet the menace of the years
Finds, and shall find, me unafraid.

It matters not how strait the gate,
How charged with punishments the scroll.
I am the master of my fate:
I am the captain of my soul.

Take command, be the captain of your soul. Revere your sleep. Got it? Good.

I recall in my own Navy days aboard a nuclear submarine that sleep was precious, as I recounted in my Introduction, yet it also seemed a luxury at times. I was always amazed to watch the skipper perform on very little sleep when we were on mission, close to the foreign navies and ports we observed. Yet, when the boat was in transit, he always managed to get better bunk time, delegating duties to the Executive Officer and the commander of the day. Operational success demanded that sleep become as important as drills, training, and preparation of all weapons, propulsion, and navigation systems. A tired crew does not integrate well with a submarine, and rest assured the art of the catnap was well practiced in all compartments. Micro-naps, or "droning" in place, were all too common.

The enemy will always attack 'sleep' and try to keep you in a sleepless state, with the goal of creating sleep deprivation. An obvious strategy, I suppose. Definitely something that Rogers' Rangers knew, and I am certain has been the case for all soldiers. Think about the role of the command in implementing a sleep readiness policy. Think about that part of you, deep within, that may be "attacking" your desire and intention to sleep.

Remember, you are in command.

What is *your* sleep policy? Essential or luxury? How much sleep is enough, at a minimum for adequate performance, and how much sleep is needed for consistent higher performance? The decision to view sleep as essential will vastly improve the quality of your daily life, your career, your relationships, your health, and your overall happiness.

The commanding officer — just as you are your own commanding officer accountable to self for performance and decisions — must make sleep a priority. The CO of a ship is responsible for the readiness of all hands. Your own readiness improves when sleep is a priority.

As the U.S. Naval Institute states for its ship captains, in an article by Captain John Cordle, USN (Retired), titled "Captain, Get Some Sleep!":

> Certainly, a CO on a ship underway must be available 24/7 for contact reports, to make critical tactical decisions, and to mentor and train the crew, but there are ways to plan ahead and set priorities.
>
> - *Set sleep goals.* The Naval Surface Forces Crew Endurance instruction requires 7 hours of sleep either in one sitting or a shorter session followed by a nap. Work this

into your plan for the day.

- *Value sleep.* Keep a routine, to include naps when appropriate.
- *Trust your crew.* Empower them to speak up when they note that you are getting tired or have been up for too long. Expect the same for them.
- *Educate yourself.* I am always amazed that intelligent, educated officers can be dismissive of the science of sleep.

I wonder how the above translates to your own life? Sleep is a valuable resource. It is time to start treating it as such.

Clearly, I am using 'military sleep' as a metaphor for your perspective on sleep, for it applies equally to your life as it does to the life of a soldier or sailor. At the very least, I wonder, as you sail your ship of life, whether you'll decide to 'rest your oars' at day's end and focus on your sleep.

While the Bud Winter technique explained in this chapter is foundational to the I Am Sleeping Now method, and you have enough to move forward, I want to say a little bit more about the military's attitudes and practices when it comes to the subject of sleep.

Hey, this is not the military, I know, but a little discipline, self-care, and personal accountability in working on habits and performance gains goes a long way. As Sam Fellman writes in *Business Insider* and at taskandpurpose.com:

> Special operation forces, who are sent on the U.S. military's most dangerous assignments, must sleep when they can and often face extreme sleep deprivation to complete their mission. Whether you're a new parent, have a stressful job or are dealing with a difficult situation, there's a lot you can learn from these elite operators.

In Fellman's article, U.S. Navy SEAL veteran Adam La Reau, co-founder of O2X Human Performance, prescribes several recommendations worth sharing.

First, he recommends having a pre-sleep game plan, confirming what this book is all about, and covered in more detail in Chapter Nine. He says to focus on "activities that will calm your nerves, maybe reading, meditation, listening to music, dimming the lights." The goal of this, by the way, is to calm the brain and avoid disrupting the circadian rhythm. Light exposure can fool your body into an awake state when sleep is the intention, pushing it away!

Secondly, La Reau recommends that you "sleep when you can" and that, "Naps are really helpful, and any sleep is better than no sleep at all." Which is good advice for the exhausted special forces operator, and for you as well, when sleep opportunities are scarce. More on napping in Chapter Six.

Also, I could save this for another chapter but let me say a little bit more here about light exposure. Speaking of light being a factor in your ability to calm your nervous system, here's what you should know, simply for the science of light's effect on the body as you evaluate and redesign your pre-sleep routine. Our mammalian brain is a pharmacy that releases chemicals and electrical signals to our body based on all sorts of stimuli. For example, facial muscles in the form of a smile cause endorphins to be released, making us feel happier. The brain knows by our smile — real or faked — that we are, or want to feel, happy.

Regarding light, your brain's hypothalamus helps regulate response to light and the subsequent arousal of the body. The hypothalamus releases the neuropeptide orexin in response to the light hitting the eyes, which then stimulates arousal, and the transition from sleep to waking then occurs. Exposure to blue light from electronics in the hours approaching sleep can delay the natural production of melatonin.

Here's the issue; electronic devices emit short-wavelength enriched light, also known as blue light. Fluorescent and LED lights can emit blue light as well. Consider blue-blocker glasses if you must expose yourself to computer monitors, smartphones, or other devices. Other than that, your new pre-sleep routine, as you slowly make changes, will manage your melatonin and orexin for you, quite naturally.

The good news is that you can interrupt old patterns, put new habits in place, and conquer this sleep issue.

According to the Sleep Foundation, as presented in the article "How Electronics Affect Sleep," at www.sleepfoundation.org, a recent survey "found that roughly four in 10 Americans bring their cell phone into bed when trying to fall asleep." (Based on my work as a clinical hypnotist, I think that number is higher!) The article goes on to state:

> Additionally, six in 10 respondents claimed to use a desktop or laptop computer within one hour of going to bed. Tempting as it might be to use your computer or phone before bed, studies have shown these devices can interfere with sleep by suppressing the production of melatonin, a natural hormone released in the evening to help you feel tired and ready for sleep. This leads to neurophysiologic arousals that increase feelings of alertness when you should be winding down instead.

As you design your new sleep routine, incorporate the above advice from the Sleep Foundation. While you are at it, give serious consideration to placing your smartphone out of reach, away from the bed. Get it out from under the pillow and off the mattress! Place it on your dresser, or some other location that's more than an arm's length away, so that you can't even be tempted to pick it up.

Remember that I said I was on a mission to help you sleep better? Well, I hope that this is all starting to make better sense for you, as you commit to taking deliberate action to take back control and start getting better, more consistent ZZZs.

Zzz-Tip: A major key to sleep improvement lies in reducing your exposure to blue light in the hours leading up to sleep time.

The discussion of light's effect on our ability to sleep is important, as Navy SEAL Adam La Reau touches upon in his article, so let me shed some more "light" on the subject. (Sorry, I could not resist the pun.)

When you are trying to invite sleep, dimming the lights is key.

Blue light is everywhere, sunlight being the main source. Limiting our exposure to light, especially indoor, man-made sources of blue light, helps the brain prepare the body for sleep by releasing more melatonin. Most notably, amounts of blue light emissions are most significant from such sources as tablets, computers, smartphones, and televisions. While the amount of blue light from these sources is far less than from sunlight, it is the cumulative effect of close proximity exposure that can impact the onset of sleep and, further, can negatively impact your eye health. Ask your eye doctor.

Be aware, however, that not all blue light is bad for you. Blue light plays an important role in helping to regulate your circadian rhythm — the body's natural system for managing the sleep and awake states. Exposure to natural sunlight during the day helps with alertness, elevates your mood, and helps with memory and cognitive functioning. Sunlight is good for you. Aside from a natural source of vitamin D, it helps you regulate melatonin. I have mentioned the circadian rhythm several times in this book. Our *circadian rhythm* occurs naturally for all humans and animals. It is an internal process that regulates the sleep–wake cycle and repeats approximately every 24 hours, based on the earth's rotation. Our circadian cycle is also affected by light, temperature, and jet lag (which zooms us to another time zone, altering our body's rhythm).

There are myriad companies offering blue-blocker glasses to protect the eyes, but the ophthalmology profession does not think they are necessary, nor are they proven effective in protecting the eyes. While the American Academy of Ophthalmology says in their report, "Should You Be Worried About Blue Light?" found at www.aao.org, that "there is no scientific evidence that blue light from digital devices causes damage to your eye," they *do* point out that exposure to blue light does impact sleep. Dr. Rahul Khurana, in the report, goes on to say, "Blue light does affect the body's circadian rhythm, our natural wake and sleep cycle. During the day, blue light wakes us up and stimulates us. But too much blue light exposure late at night from your phone, tablet, or computer can make it harder to get to sleep."

As you focus on returning to your natural ability to sleep well again, make note of your habits and what you are willing to change. Additionally, in the above report, Dr. Khurana recommends "that you try to limit your screen time in the two to three hours before you go to bed. You can also try nighttime settings on your devices to minimize blue light exposure in the evenings." Sage advice. I say it's best to limit exposure and get into a new pre-sleep routine. This will help your brain's pineal gland release melatonin as you use your full mind and body's power to bring sleep to your bedside!

If you need further proof of blue light's negative impact on sleep, just check out the research article from the PNAS (Proceedings of the National Academy of Sciences of the United States of America), titled "Evening use of light-emitting eReaders negatively affects sleep, circadian timing, and next-morning alertness," available on PubMed or at the source, www.pnas.org/content/112/4/1232.

Some of the salient points taken directly from the report, verbatim, which impact your sleep mission:

In the past 50 years, there has been a decline in average sleep duration and quality, with adverse consequences on general health. A representative survey of 1,508 American adults recently revealed that 90% of Americans used some type of electronics at least a few nights per week within 1 h before bedtime. Mounting evidence from countries around the world shows the negative impact of such technology use on sleep. This negative impact on sleep may be due to the short-wavelength-enriched light emitted by these electronic devices, given that artificial-light exposure has been shown experimentally to produce alerting effects, suppress melatonin, and phase-shift the biological clock.

The use of electronic devices for reading, communication, and entertainment has greatly increased in recent years. Greater portability, convenience, and ease of access to reading materials in electronic form add to the popularity of these devices. The use of light-emitting devices immediately before bedtime is a concern because light is the most potent environmental signal that impacts the human circadian clock and may therefore play a role in perpetuating sleep deficiency.

We found that, compared with reading a printed book in reflected light, reading a light-emitting eBook in the hours before bedtime decreased subjective sleepiness, decreased EEG delta/theta activity, and suppressed the late evening rise of pineal melatonin secretion during the time that the book was being read. We also found that, compared with reading a printed book, reading an LE-eBook in the hours before bedtime lengthened sleep latency; delayed the phase of the endogenous circadian pacemaker that drives the timing of daily rhythms of melatonin secretion, sleep propensity, and REM sleep propensity; and impaired morning alertness.

The decreased sleepiness before bedtime and longer sleep latency we observed in the LE-eBook condition is likely due to both an acute alerting effect of light and a delay of the circadian timing system. Suppression of melatonin by exposure to evening light may be an underlying mechanism by which light acutely increases alertness.

I recommend you make a note to read this report later, if you want to more deeply understand the science of managing your circadian rhythm and the impact of your self-sabotaging habits of melatonin suppression. For now, read a paper book instead of an eBook late at night. Reading with reflected light is better, near sleep time, than from back-lit devices.

Zzz-Tip: In the shift to this new work-from-home paradigm that we're currently experiencing, two noteworthy trends can also impact our ability to sleep well. The low cost of high-quality monitors means that many at-home workers are using dual screens for their computer work. Dual screens late in the evening may further delay sleep onset when we eventually hit the pillow. Additionally, online video conferencing and meetings, webinars, et al, are stimulating our minds (and that pineal gland) late in the evening, delaying the release of melatonin. Turn down the brightness, limit late-night exposure.

The Pineal Gland? What's That?

The pineal gland is located deep within the brain, between the left and right hemispheres, in the middle of the head. (It holds calcified structures called *Corpora arenacea*, also referred to as "brain sand," which radiographers use as a marker on X-ray images to locate the brain's center.) In terms of understanding the body, the pineal gland was one of the last organs of the brain to be discovered. At the time, 17th-century French philosopher René Descartes, in his books *Treatise of Man* and *Passions of the Soul* (two famous books on the subject of pineal neuropsychology and neurophysiology), had claimed that the soul was located in the pineal gland, perhaps because it was the center of the brain. Exploring Descartes is fun for the philosophy-minded, but it would be a tangential journey for the adventurous and a sidestep to our mission here, in this book. Descartes, St. Augustine, and St. Thomas Aquinas seemed to be on course for figuring out the mind–body–soul connection in their time. All good reading — after you have completed your sleep mastery skills. Who knows? Maybe Descartes can lull you to sleep after a few pages!

One of the functions of the pineal gland, a relatively recent discovery in terms of brain research, is to produce melatonin. Much is still not fully understood about the pineal gland, but it is scientifically accepted that it plays a key role in setting sleep patterns and the awake–asleep cycles of the body. Melatonin is a hormone secreted by the pineal gland, regulating the body's internal clock — the circadian timing system in the body. It is secreted more so when it is dark, pointing to its role in sleep.

Let's not overthink the importance of the pineal gland. You and your primary care physician can determine appropriate next steps, as can your sleep doctor. Low-dose melatonin supplements may be beneficial, but since I make no claims to the efficacy of any medications or supplements, consult your doctor if you have questions — and I do not mean Dr. Google!

Zzz-TIP: Practice the sleep techniques that Bud Winter developed for the military in World War II. The concepts and methods apply to all humans. You may not be under the same pressures as combat military personnel, but when sleep comes, or is sought, you ought to feel now like you are able to take control of your mind and body — and the physical and mental relaxation will unlock your success.

Before you turn to Chapter Five, pause for a moment and reflect on your reaction to the information presented in this current chapter.

- What lessons will you take from the military's success in combatting sleep issues?
- Can you begin to feel a sense of calm and inner peace as you focus on and take control of your sleep situation?
- What changes are you already contemplating in your relationship with sleep?

Okay, that was a lot of information discussed. I am ready to turn the page. I know you are as well!

CHAPTER FIVE

Take Charge of Your Sleep with Self-Hypnosis!

"Sex and sleep alone make me conscious that I am a mortal."
—Alexander the Great

Alexander the Great also said, "There is nothing impossible to him who will try!"

I know that you succeed at whatever you put your mind to, and not because I say so, but because when you recall something you really set out to accomplish and succeeded, it felt great. Now with that in mind, just imagine for a moment how it will feel with your sleep goals realized. Own it. Focus on it. I did say at the top of this book that there is no trying, only doing, or not doing. Well, you are here, still reading, and in my mind, that's doing!

We're going to move from *trying* to sleep better, to simply sleeping better. There is a huge difference. Make it a self-fulfilling prophecy.

Keep reading!

As you create your new relationship with sleep, which is the true underlying goal of your journey, I encourage you to revisit the questions presented at the end of Chapter One. As you reread them, you may notice that you are beginning to make a shift, with a feeling of both hope and determination. You are, indeed, on a journey back to sleep mastery.

As you might surmise at this point, falling and staying asleep is primarily about having the right mindset about sleep. Hopefully, this book is helping you make a shift that makes sleep such a matter-of-fact, expected reality that soon you will simply accept this new you who is emerging. I am confident in your ability to take back control, and in doing so, take back control of other aspects of your life as well! Observe, as you awaken to that phenomenon.

Let's talk about hypnosis. I have yet to see it discussed in any of the various books about sleep on the market today. They dance around the topic, because it is either innocently overlooked, misunderstood, or feared because of its true, natural, and proven success in helping to easily resolve and/or make accelerated progress toward one's intentions. In other words, it's been omitted from the discussion at large. After all, the hypnosis solution does little to create sales of sleep devices, mattresses, or medications. Recall, as I mentioned earlier, the sleep industry is a $30B market, and you may be seeing an explosion of sleep-related products competing for your attention.

Hypnosis, however, is quite effective in treating sleep, much the same way as it is likewise used to help people stop smoking — to communicate with the subconscious mind and offer suggestions that support the desire. Within my profession, we know it works. It's driven by intentions, motivation, and a determination to enjoy the benefits of your intentions as if they were already realized. It's called *future pacing*, and works by visualizing the outcome, and connecting to the feeling of that outcome as if it has already happened. The body, and subsequent actions it takes, will follow what it believes in the mind to be true.

Meditation and relaxation are discussed in many other circles, as they should be, and they are cousins in this self-help category of personal improvement. Hypnosis adds to these modalities with an intention and opens the mind to hearing and accepting appropriate suggestions for the mind, body, and yes, even the soul.

Hypnosis is an evidence-based strategy for improving sleep. It is well proven and supported by numerous studies and is documented through antiquity, long before the word "hypnosis" was coined. Hypnosis is not putting a person to sleep, as some might believe, although it *can* be sleep-like, especially with deep hypnosis or somnambulism (a state similar to what sleepwalkers experience). There are various depth levels of hypnosis, but for our purpose of sleep mastery, a very light self-hypnotic trance is all that is needed.

Hypnosis can be achieved in the awake or conscious state, too, while fully alert, as we are always in a trance state anyway. It's true. When we are focused on a singular point of concentration we are, indeed, in a hypnotic or trance-like state, for instance. There's also something called conversational hypnosis, utilizing specific language patterns and imagery to communicate with the mind by tapping into the emotions of the individual. It is used in the clinical setting, in sales, and in marketing. It's used by any skilled influence and persuasion expert. Car salespeople study this. National brands use hypnosis in their advertising.

Hypnosis Defined

There are many different definitions of hypnosis. I like to keep it simple. I tell my clients that hypnosis is, when you boil it down to its essence, defined as "a heightened state of focused attention, awareness, and concentration," as controlled by the client. We use it to create a state of intentional absorption, focused on an intention. I point out to my clients that their subconscious mind is a vast resource of wisdom and experience, and they can speak to and access their powerful mind in hypnosis.

Beyond my definition above, let me offer a few other insights to help you see the real value of using hypnosis as a tool for behavioral change, coping with stress and anxiety, healing, and in dealing with certain mental health conditions such as PTSD, and fears and phobias (as affirmed by the Mayo Clinic on their web page about Hypnosis). Hypnosis is a trance-like condition in which people experience increased attention, concentration, and suggestibility. We use it to help set the conscious mind aside so that direct communication with our subconscious is possible. In hypnosis we can allow suggestions designed for our highest and best to be embraced and accepted as it relates to our intention.

Dr. Richard Nongard, President of the International Certification Board of Clinical Hypnotherapy, offers this definition: "Hypnosis is a state of absorption into a powerful ideas or resources states that we can use to make change. It is not something that happens to us, but something we do or generate from within ourselves."

Further rounding out a definition of hypnosis, although I think you've got it already, HMI (Hypnosis Motivation Institute), a nationally accredited college of hypnotherapy, offers this: "Hypnosis is an altered state of consciousness which results in an increased receptiveness and response to suggestion. While associated with relaxation, hypnosis is an escape from an overload of message units, resulting in relaxation. Hypnosis can be triggered naturally from environmental stimuli as well as purposefully from an operator, often referred to as a hypnotist."

I would add that the hypnotist is a guide in the process, which you control, leading to the fact that all hypnosis is self-hypnosis anyway. This book, and the I Am Sleeping Now method, are all about teaching you to be that self-directed guide when the intention is to go to sleep! In other words, you are becoming your own hypnotist, as both the suggester and the suggestee! Yes, indeed, you can take charge of your mind and condition yourself to sleep well again.

Self-hypnosis is simply, as I see it, a self-directed way to utilize your trance state for an intended purpose, such as feeding your mind a specific autosuggestion, program your mind with greater positivity, focus on an issue or situation with greater clarity, or to "install" an affirmation. Professional hypnotists use self-hypnosis, as do athletes, businesspeople, and people of all ages and walks of life to make progress toward their goal or to simply live a happier, more fulfilled, and empowered life. Think of it as a powerful mind-tool for accelerating your progress toward a goal — any goal.

By reading this book, you are learning self-hypnosis to help you sleep. It will all come together. Now, with the idea of self-hypnosis introduced, I want to share a few additional strategies that may contribute to your sleep experience.

Invoking the Relaxation Response

The relaxation response is included here because I want you to master it. It is key to your consistently improving sleep experience, as it is useful during your pre-sleep rituals and when you crawl into bed. Sorry, I know I've mentioned the importance of relaxation previously, but it bears repeating and I cannot underscore it enough. Allow me to go into it in a little more detail here, if you will, and don't be at all surprised if I bring the subject of relaxation up again later on in the book as well.

Fight, flight, or freeze! These responses are our survival instincts, coded into our genes and passed down to us by our ancestors. If there were a tiger at the door (or at the entrance to our cave), for instance, roaring and banging to get in, when presented with the tiger we are either going to freeze, run, or stand and fight the animal.

As *Harvard Health* explains, "First described by Dr. Walter B. Cannon at Harvard Medical School in the 1920s, the fight-or-flight response evolved as a survival mechanism. When we encounter a life-threatening situation, a surge of stress hormones prepares us to fight or to flee." It's an automatic response that causes temporary stress. Our body reacts to what we are sensing, thinking, and feeling, and responds. Our heart beats faster, muscles contract, adrenaline flows, arteries constrict, and we are ready to take one of those three survival responses. Sometimes, that stress response lingers. Usually, it subsides as the danger fades, but sometimes we cannot turn it off without conscious intervention. Sometimes the stress or anxiety 'program' keeps playing and we forget to realize we can turn it off.

We can calm the stress response, however, by consciously reversing the body's reaction to the perceived feelings of danger. Dr. Herbert Benson, in his 1975 book *The Relaxation Response*, taught the modern world how to do just this, and his Benson-Henry Institute for Mind Body Medicine at Massachusetts

General Hospital has been focused on the science and methods of deep relaxation. Dr. Benson, one of the world's first Western physicians to bring spirituality and mind–body healing into medicine, coined the term "relaxation response" in a 1974 article in the medical journal *Psychiatry*. At that time, he noted that such practices as Zen meditation, yoga, repetitive prayer, progressive muscle relaxation, and even hypnosis could invoke measurable physiological changes. Relaxation was measurable. In fact, this author (yours truly, Bob Martel) recently underwent electromyographic nerve testing (EMG) for a pinched nerve and was able to use self-hypnosis to show the neurologist that the relaxation response I consciously triggered had removed the measurable muscle tension in my arm. Ah, the power of the mind!

Using this relaxation technique will prepare you for better sleep. The relaxation response is defined as "the response that is the opposite of the fight-or-flight or stress response." Based on widely known practices that have been used for millennia, the relaxation response is very similar in many ways to prayer, meditation, and repetitive motion techniques such as those referred to as bilateral stimulation.

Eliciting the relaxation response takes only a few moments, and builds resiliency in mind and body, helps the immune system, and creates a feeling of control over emotions. And it also, in plain words, just makes you feel so damn relaxed!

When we practice the relaxation response, which you are about to learn, the body becomes more physiologically relaxed. Blood pressure is lowered, blood flow is increased, oxygen to the blood is optimized, and hormones return to normal levels. Over the past few decades, as Benson explains in his latest book on the subject, *The Relaxation Revolution*, the technique has been proven effective in many ways, including lowering blood pressure, as cited in his 1974 study published in *The Lancet*, and in aiding in reducing or eliminating insomnia.

The relaxation response is easy to learn and practice. Too many meditation gurus complicate the process. It is merely a matter of breathing and focusing, and can be accomplished in a matter of moments. With the addition of an anchor or two to connect your intention to a feeling, you can shift from the stress–fear state to a calm and relaxed state, invoking the exact opposite of the stress response. Keep it simple and you cannot fail at this!

Practicing the relaxation response, on a regular basis, is transformational. It is a time set aside for you to shift from the busy pace of life, to pause and be present with yourself, sitting quietly and still. This allows your mind and body to restore, focusing simply on the breath, or on a selected word such as "calm" or "relaxed."

Now, with that said, realize that there is no one way to practice the relaxation response successfully. It's all about focus and breaking the train of everyday thought to, in Benson's words, "evoke this physiological state." Before I walk you through the technique, let me share a few examples of people deliberately immersed in the relaxation response:

- The bingo hall filled with people dabbing their sheets, some with their good luck charms and trolls by their side, moving their arms in unison to the caller's numbers, focused intently on calling "bingo!" when their number is shouted out. They are in the zone.

- The person practicing yoga or Tai Chi in a class or in front of the TV with their at-home video classes. They are in the zone, too, focused on the movements and the instruction from their teacher.

- The person practicing their musical instrument or singing in the shower. Focused, relaxed, in the zone.

- The athlete on the gridiron, the ballfield, the tennis court, or the lacrosse field — focused on relaxing into the process of enjoying playing their chosen sport. In the zone.

- The person feeling stress and anxiety who can practice what you will learn next to consciously invoke Dr. Benson's technique. You'll be in the zone, and further, you'll be able to instantly call up that relaxed state using your new self-hypnosis techniques, too!

Here is one technique for invoking the relaxation response. It is based on Benson's basic guidance, and it can be the foundation for innumerous strategies to relax deeply. Paraphrasing his explanation:

1) Select a repetitive thought upon which you can focus, while disregarding other thoughts when they come to mind. It's easier than you might think, and just requires a little mind conditioning. I am confident you'll get the hang of it.

    a. Let's use the words "calm" and "relax."

    b. You could also choose a word like "peace" or "love," as Benson also suggests.

    c. You could choose a faith-based anchor word or phrase such as "Jesus," "Hail Mary/Ave Maria," "Shalom," or other peaceful spiritual words for your faith, or phrases that reset your mind in this direction.

2) As Benson suggests, if other thoughts float to the surface while attempting to relax and focus, simply say "oh well," and without judgment or criticism, be aware of it, and let it float away as you bring your attention back to your intention.

3) Sit comfortably, close your eyes, and take a deep relaxing breath, the best breath you can take. In through your nose, hold it for a few seconds, and exhale through your mouth. Now, again, and as you do so, say your chosen word or phrase to yourself silently as you breathe in again, and exhale again, being sure to take a full belly breath and pausing before you exhale, allowing for a full exchange of oxygen into your lungs, and carbon dioxide out.

4) Take a moment to double-check your comfort position. Relax all the muscles in your body. Your feet, up your legs to your hips, further up, up, to your core, your neck and shoulders, your arms. Let your entire face and jaw relax. Breathe again, saying your chosen word or phrase.

5) Expect and anticipate other thoughts to emerge. Simply usher them along and stay focused on your breathing.

6) Breathe and relax for four to five minutes.

7) Now, with that relaxation response in place, keep your eyes closed as you begin to emerge now, allowing your regular thoughts to return. And, then, slowly open your eyes.

8) Sit for a moment with eyes open before getting back up.

Practice relaxation daily. I cannot stress this enough. Decide it's a skill worth living, as it could indeed change the very course of your life. Have courage enough to go there!

It is best if you can find a small bit of time in the morning, before breakfast perhaps, for five minutes or so, after dinner for five minutes, and also for a few minutes during your new pre-sleep habitual rituals you are embracing on this journey. Later, we'll talk about anchoring your relaxed state to a cue that you can use throughout your day, and prior to sleep.

As I mentioned, and as Benson emphasizes, there are many ways to accomplish relaxation. For our purposes, the above works quite well. It is something I teach all my clinical hypnosis clients to do! Now it's your turn to practice it! Dr. Benson's original book, *The Relaxation Response*, and his newer book, *Relaxation Revolution: The Science and Genetics of Mind Body Healing*, are valuable resources and both belong on your bookshelf. Make a note of it, as I want to do my best and stay on track.

I hope I am giving you enough of a foundation to see that you have more control over this than you first thought possible, and that you can go quickly and easily to sleep using my I AM SLEEPING NOW method.

This is a good place to tell you about Martha, one of my clients. She came to me for some clinical hypnosis work that we did together, to help her take back control of her anxiety and stress. Martha was 75 years old at the time. She was always worrying about the future, and most of those worries and fears were all quite irrational, and she knew that, but she just did not know how to make the shift she so wanted. She confided to me that throughout her entire life, she had always been anxious.

Now, imagine Martha, sitting in my office. A bit anxious about hypnosis because it was, for her, a new and unfamiliar experience. We did a little deep breathing, and I showed her a few fun

81

hypnotic phenomena to build her confidence in her decision to make the appointment. Then, I said to Martha, *"Martha, take another nice breath… a belly breath… that's right… and as you exhale, I want you to simply say the word 'calm' as you decide to let yourself relax…"*

Well, the word *relax* was all she needed to hear! She sat up in the chair, opened her eyes, glared at me and said, "Relaxation is such a waste of time! Who has time for this?"

Now, relaxation is not entirely necessary for success with hypnosis, but in a clinical setting it is very useful and quite therapeutic, as you just learned from Dr. Benson, right? I had to think fast. "Martha," I said. "What if I told you that relaxation was a key strategy to help you realize your intentions? That it was important to the progress we were going to make?"

Bingo! She was excited to experience deep relaxation, and she did. When our session was over and she emerged from hypnosis, she was crying. She said she wished she had learned to relax 40 years earlier in life because, had that been the case, her life would have been so very much different today. I think I shed a tear that day with her.

Let's Get Your Mind, Body, Spirit, and Heart in Alignment

Your sleep mastery skills are centered on having a coherent brain and heart, which simply means being in a state of alignment or integration with the intentions of your mind, body, and spirit. Your subconscious can detect this alignment and help you move toward realizing any intention, including sleep. When our thoughts are aligned with our true intentions, and our heart and brain are thus in harmony, our entire body responds.

When we are in alignment, with a congruent heart and brain, we positively impact our physical health, we are more resilient because our sense of conviction and our immune system are stronger, our energy improves, and we have a more positive outlook on life with a better sense of self-control and determination. In a state of coherence, we live more authentically in the moment, connected to our true self, living our life deliberately, peacefully, and naturally, with less stress and more happiness day to day. We achieve coherence when the brain, which is the primary nerve center for thoughts, emotions, and decisions, works "hand in glove" with the heart (which is also a center for emotions), and also with our body as a whole. It is that harmony that occurs between our mind, body, and spirit — a harmonious state that we can create within ourselves through meditation, relaxation, and self-hypnosis.

"Coherence is the state when the heart, mind, and emotions are in energetic alignment and cooperation," HeartMath Institute director of research Dr. Rollin McCraty explains. "It is a state that builds resiliency — personal energy is accumulated, not wasted — leaving more energy to manifest intentions and harmonious outcomes."

The heart is usually left out of the discussion of mind–body–spirit development and alignment. As the HeartMath Institute, a non-profit researching this coherence, states on their website:

> Adding heart translates into increased care and genuine connection with others and harmonizes the resistance between our own mind and heart. Adding heart is especially about practicing kindness and compassion, along with forgiveness and latitude in our interactions. Adding heart increases the love flowing through our system, which can play a large part in solving the collective challenges of these transitional times.

Heart–brain coherence is worthy of your further examination, as an important piece of the overall sleep puzzle. (When you go to www.iamsleepingnow.com you can get on the email list, if you'd like, and can grab additional resources which will say more about HeartMath.)

Here's what I would like you to know for our purposes in sleep mastery:

- Science says that our heart produces an electromagnetic field, affected by our emotional states, which have an effect on the communication to the brain.

- Negative emotions and stress, as you might guess, cause disorder and inhibit clear communications. Our ability to reason, to see with greater clarity, recall, and make good decisions are all negatively impacted as a result.

- The reverse is true as well: *Positive* emotions have a tremendous impact on how we see the world (so we can act in a more deliberate manner).

While the heart is a source of energy feeding the brain, the brain also feeds the entire body. It is a pharmacy releasing chemicals, accessed and triggered by a host of sources, including emotions, intentions, actions, and decisions we make. It senses muscle position, as in the face for example. A smiling face will cause endorphins to be released. So, as you go to bed, in your new pre-sleep routine, try to smile for a few minutes before slipping under the sheets. Endorphins will flow. Force the smile if necessary!

Creating heart–brain coherence will change your life. Heart–brain coherence is best achieved when our actions move us toward progress in realizing our intentions — mind, body, spirit, and heart all "rowing together" to make an intention a reality. Our body can sense the alignment of our intentions and our actions. If the intention is real but the actions that support that intention fall short or are misguided, the rhythm of the heart is out of synch with the brain and may be a source of ongoing stress. The subconscious mind knows when you really want what you say you want, and it's looking for congruence of thoughts, feelings, and behaviors. With alignment, your mind, body, and spirit will deliver what is in your power to control. Sleep is a good example.

Imagine or envision you sleeping well again in the very near future. Let that be your intention. On a multisensory level, experience what it will be like to enjoy rising refreshed and ready to greet the day. It will feel wonderful. Pause for a moment to amplify the positive emotion that comes from picturing this in your mind. Connect with that inner vision as if you are already enjoying it! (What you picture, imagine, and focus upon is what comes true!)

With coherence, the heart and brain develop a harmonious rhythm, working as designed, in a calm and relaxed manner, to help you take your life in the direction you want it to go. The heart responds in a different, healthier way, all quite measurable. Our energy levels are better, as with coherence there is no wasted heart–brain energy. Our internal systems are operating at optimal performance, as designed, when peace and harmony fill our hearts. When negative emotions are amplified or when people are living in a state of fear or anger it causes the heart to beat out of rhythm.

Each one of us can train ourselves to increase our heart–mind coherence. Guided meditation or, quite simply, self-hypnosis, helps to create heart and brain coherence. You can learn how to calm your mind and body, and how to overcome your past and create a new future for yourself. Your new tomorrow starts tonight, with a better night's sleep. You have the power to shift your perspective, and become your new future self — a better sleeper — simply by connecting to that future self in this present moment.

Let me teach you now, how to quickly create a more coherent heart–mind state in about 60 seconds. It's a pretty simple yet powerful process you can practice anytime throughout the day to keep yourself calm and coherent. As you practice this technique, you'll see how it fits in with your self-hypnotic power naps as well as with your pre-sleep routine. (More on hypnotic power naps in the next chapter.) Heart–brain coherence is the body's natural desired state, and is an essential condition that invites sleep, naturally.

Here are the steps to creating coherence almost instantly. Use them to tap into your creativity and be ready to perform at your best:

• Without too much effort, summon up an intentional positive feeling, perhaps an act of compassion or self-compassion, kindness, care of others or self, or a sense of gratitude and peace. Smile, inward or outwardly. Putting your facial muscles in a smile position releases endorphins, making you feel happier.

- Focus your attention on the physical area around your heart. If privacy is available, you may even want to place one or both hands over your heart as you take a relaxing deep breath. Close your eyes if you'd like, but it's not necessary. You can do this in your (parked) car before walking into the office, at a meeting, in a chair at the beach, or even just prior to bed. Anywhere at all! Just keep your attention focused on your heart.

- Continue to breathe in a deep, relaxed manner, taking a full belly breath, or diaphragmatic breath. Use your wonderful imagination and pretend, as you breathe using all five lobes of your lungs (the left lung has two, and the right lung has three!), that it seems like you are breathing from your heart — a true heart-centered breath. As you inhale, think *"calm,"* and as you exhale think *"relax,"* and notice the soothing rhythm of your breathing. Notice the natural rhythm of your breathing and enjoy it. Magical.

- Turn on that summoned positive feeling now, connecting with a time when you experienced love in your heart, or when you felt gratitude or deep appreciation for something you experienced, or, simply take yourself to that special and safe, happy place within yourself. Continue to breathe and relax.

The benefits of practicing this are limitless. Your mind, body, and spirit will begin to love this special gift you give to your own heart and the change within you will be amazing. Blood flow increases. Blood pressure decreases. More oxygen is delivered to every cell in your body. This is also an excellent technique for helping to lower stress and eliminate anxiety.

Shifting to a life filled with gratitude helps improve the overall quality of daily living, and it helps us to more easily fall and stay asleep. When we direct our attention to more positive and realistic thoughts, taking stock of our gifts, talents, and blessings, peace of mind comes more easily — which in turn helps us sleep better.

When you say to yourself, *"I can't sleep,"* you are creating heart–mind incoherence. However, when you shift that inner dialogue to, *"I am training my mind and body to sleep well again,"* or words to that effect, and you connect to that vision, you are creating coherence, and lowering your stress levels. Breathing to relax also causes coherence. Choosing to watch and control your inner self-talk and your breathing will help you condition yourself to easily fall and stay asleep!

Remember, the subconscious mind is a habit mind, programmed by you! This entire book is centered on resetting your subconscious programming in regard to sleep. It is about you deciding to take action to change habits — your habitual rituals, as I call them — whether actions, inactions, or thoughts. You are reading this book consciously, feeding your mind new knowledge and insights (which is good!), but change requires a little something more. Your own subconscious programming may be at the heart of what is keeping you from getting what you want! New thoughts, with mental rehearsal and visions of the outcome already achieved (better sleep), will lead to that new you emerging as you embrace and apply what you discover about yourself here in these pages.

You must feel excited and empowered, filled with positivity, I hope! And I know it may be a bit difficult to imagine, but as you embrace all I've said, or at least some of it, you are fast becoming more connected with yourself, and with family, friends, co-workers and others, and with the world!

Zzz-Tip: So, you can see your sleep strategy building upon relaxation, self-hypnosis, and the alignment of mind, body, and spirit. Everyone loves to talk about mind–body–spirit. Draw a small triangle off in the margin somewhere. At the top of the triangle, label that with "M" for Mind. Do the same at the other corners, with "B" for Body and "S" for Spirit. Leave enough space to draw a small heart inside the triangle. Now draw a line from the mind directly to the heart, connecting the two together. Start to envision your mind, body, spirit, and heart working together for your absolute highest and best. You see, the quality of your sleep and the ease of entering this inescapable and hopefully welcoming realm are directly related to the peace, joy, and tranquility in your life, which is determined by so many factors, including your kindness and compassion as a person, your ability to forgive, the gratitude you celebrate in daily life, and your connection to your Divine purpose. This peace within, this living authentically, this congruence, balance, and alignment, all help you sleep soundly every night! I hope you agree — because it's true!

When you do this, when you are courageous enough to get into alignment — (it's a process!) — you begin to chart a new course, a new destiny. Living a heart-centered life helps you sleep better! Taking control of your emotions, and choosing happiness, are key.

Kokoro, Kaizen, Ikigai, and the Welcoming Path

Almost sounds as if I might be launching into a story, or a joke, doesn't it? Okay, so Kokoro, Kaizen, and Ikigai all walk into a bar, right? Bartender says...

Alright, all silliness aside, the discussion of these three ideas may fall slightly outside the scope of developing your sleep mastery skills. Or then again perhaps not. Allow me to briefly introduce these three important concepts to you, if you'd be so kind, and I'll lead into it by relating something personal.

I raised three sons, all fine young men. I told each of them two things. First, always be there for your brothers. And secondly, find out what makes you happy in life and go do it; find a way to make a good living doing what truly makes you happy. I told each of them to find their *ikigai*, which they did. They found their appreciation for *kaizen* also, developing a better sense of self-worth in the process, as well as embracing *kokoro*.

Let me explain, as these are likely three unfamiliar terms.

生き甲斐

Ikigai (also *ikigagi*) is a Japanese concept for our *raison d'être*, or reason for being — our purpose in life. When we know, are connected to, and are living our purpose, we are happier. File this idea. Go look for your *ikigai* later, as it is a life-long process for

88

some, and an instant revelation for others. For now, know that it's a key to happiness and, you guessed it, better sleep. Alignment of your mind, body, spirit, and heart, by the way, also means alignment with God, or your higher source if you prefer.

In my hypnosis practice I help my clients find their *ikigai* so they can once again feel that *joie de vivre* — their joy for life! It is a process, a journey of self-discovery, awareness, and reflection with intention, and includes several factors.

To summarize it here for you, *ikigai* is, as described over at happiness.com:

> [T]he passion and talent we have, that gives meaning to our days and drives us to share the best of ourselves with the world. *Ikigai* is an attitude towards life, a way of finding our optimal activities in life, and a set of characteristics that can create meaning and happiness in life. *Ikigai* is found at the intersection where passion, mission, vocation, and profession meet.

Among the concepts of *ikigai* are:
- Nurturing good, healthy habits.
- Finding the flow of daily living in an active lifestyle.
- Slowing down, living an unhurried life, and eliminating worry.
- Nurturing relationships and being present with people.
- Maintaining an optimistic view and sharing a smile.

For our goals of helping to invite and enjoy sleep each night, remember it is important to know your purpose in life. Go on that journey after reading this book.

改善

Kaizen is the Japanese word for continuous improvement or change for the better. The concept is best known as it is applied to business, with a commitment to improvement from all levels of a company — from the CEO to the workers on an assembly line or service delivery team. Just as in business, there is always room for personal improvement, too. Incremental changes add up and make a significant positive impact. With greater awareness, as the *kaizen* philosophical belief ascribes, everything can be improved. It is not about perfection; rather, it is about positive change.

I offer the Japanese concept of *kaizen* here as a tool for continuous self-improvement in your daily life, and especially as it relates to improvement in your pre-sleep habitual rituals.

I wonder, as you inform your mind to see, what greater awareness you will begin to develop as you focus on your intention to bring sleep to your pillow? Hmmm. I wonder, too, what incremental changes you will make as you shift and prepare better for a restful sleep.

Kokoro is a common Japanese word meaning inseparable heart and mind working together, driven by our intentions. Sounds a lot like heart–brain coherence, and it has a similar meaning. According to my handy Japanese–English dictionary, *kokoro* refers to all human activities affecting the outside world through intention, emotion, and intellect. All in one word, it connects our physical heart, our mind, and the essence of our being.

"*Kokoro* is well understood in Japanese, but difficult to explain in English," says Yoshikawa Sakiko, director of Kyoto University's Kokoro Research Center. Conceptually, it unites the notions of heart, mind, and spirit; it sees these three elements as being indivisible from one other. "For example, if we say, 'She has a good *kokoro*,' it means heart and spirit and soul and mind all together." One of the problems of discussing *kokoro* in English is that by linking the words heart and spirit and mind with "*and*," we imply divisions that simply don't exist in Japanese. But in this Eastern culture, the three aren't intrinsically linked as one; rather, they *are* one. Inseparable. They function together.

So, you may be thinking that *ikigai*, *kaizen*, and *kokoro* have absolutely nothing to do with your sleep mastery skills. Think again. *Kokoro* suggests the interconnectedness of everything.

Kaizen suggests a commitment to continuous self-improvement and to processes or routines that affect our life. *Ikigai* suggests that in finding your purpose, you will be happier, experience the benefit of a more fulfilling day, and thus, hit the pillow ready for sleep.

Emotional Intelligence and Maturity

Let's add your emotional self-control to the skills mastery mix.

Congruence, which we've been discussing, also enables more emotional self-control. And with greater mental and emotional discipline, we begin to stop running from our emotions, using various distracting behaviors. We face them, we welcome them, and we manage them. We can control our emotions when we want to do so. Fear leaves us, for example, or becomes the motivation for change. Our emotions exist to help us respond to the sensations, thoughts, and feelings we experience. Emotional intelligence allows us to bring the best possible perspective to a situation by controlling our responses to triggers.

When we sleep well, we are sharper during the day. When we are sharper during the day, we tend to sleep better because of the quality of our decisions and the impact of emotional responses as we move through the day. Make sense? It's an important correlation, and is food for thought for us here. For now, be aware that developing better emotional skills fits in with your strategy toward enjoying better sleep and awake time. *Kaizen*, *ikigai*, and *kokoro* at work in your daily life will help you sleep better and better, and aid in your emotional self-control.

Let's talk a bit more about emotional intelligence and its relation to your sleep mastery.

Emotional intelligence is defined, primarily, as the ability to perceive emotions in oneself and others, and the ability to choose the most effective response in various situations. There is a strong connection between emotional intelligence and quality of sleep that we enjoy, and sleep plays an important role in managing emotions. This is well-researched and proven. In the field of neurophysiology, sleep scientists recommend a solid eight-hour sleep session, for the purpose of maximizing REM sleep, which allows for clearer thinking.

Have you ever been told, or suggested to someone, "Why don't you sleep on it and make a decision in the morning"? Of course. There's wisdom in that advice. Here's the connection:

- We are more empathetic and compassionate of others, and we also tend not to be quite as hard on ourselves when we sleep well. Our inner critic tends to overdramatize what is really happening in the moment when we are sleep-deprived.

- Sleep enables us to be more elastic and more empathetic, meaning we can better sense what is really going on around us. Lack of sleep impacts our ability to accurately read facial expressions — the non-verbal communication mechanism that telegraphs what a person is thinking and feeling. Misreads lead to incorrect interpretations and likely misdeeds.

- Our creative juices flow better with a good night's rest, or even in bursts after a quick nap (as Salvador Dali, for one, perfected). Creativity fosters flexibility and adaptability to given situations, offering clarity of mind for exploring perhaps otherwise unforeseen options or opportunities. Again, more on napping in Chapter Six.

The link between sleep and emotional intelligence does not infer that intelligent people sleep more soundly. It does mean, however, that those who have a better grasp at managing their emotional state and responses to what triggers a behavior (or not) tend to sleep better. Sleep and emotional intelligence are intertwined, each influencing the other. A sleep-deprived person experiences decreased emotional intelligence as well as decreased critical thinking or learning skills.

Some other key aspects in regard to emotional intelligence, worthy of your exploration, include:

- Intra-personal functioning, meaning how well you regard yourself and, quite frankly, how good you are to yourself, or not. This is important. You are worthy and deserving, and it may be time for you to be a little bit better to yourself.

In my hypnosis practice I help my clients reconnect or develop new attitudes and beliefs regarding self-love, self-respect, self-compassion, self-actualization, and self-care. Each can make a difference in one's ability to fall and stay asleep as they influence your life's daily experience.

- Can you handle things without going off the rails? Stress-management skills are essential. I teach my clients to condition themselves to become and stay calm, relaxed, and in control of their emotions in any given situation, using breathing, anchoring, and self-talk to control their emotions, feelings, and actions. Stress reduction is essential, too, and this chapter should help in that regard.

- Outlook, perspectives, and behavioral coping skills. Are you able to shift to a positive outlook, with consideration for blessings, gratitude, and acknowledgment of your special God-given gifts? Doing so will help you sleep better as you connect with the authentic self, connected to purpose and living in the present moment. It helps you hit the pillow with a clear, calm mind, ready for slumber.

The relationship between emotional intelligence and sleep quality is becoming better understood. Without going into the particular details of it, one individual study of 377 students undertaken at Ferdowsi University in Iran, under the auspices of Tehran University, concluded:

> The optimal sleep quality can be related to higher emotional intelligence. Amongst the two sleep quality components, the total sleep quality had a stronger relationship with emotional intelligence. It may be inferred that to increase student productivity, emotion-focused psychological interventions should focus on utilization, appraisal, and regulation of emotions.

This study mapping the correlation between sleep quality and emotional intelligence, or emotional maturity, used two primary instruments — the self-reporting Pittsburgh Sleep Quality Index (PSQI), which was developed by the University of Pittsburgh (www.sleep.pitt.edu), and the Emotional Intelligence Scale (EIS). In addition to these, you may also find the Schutte Self-Report Emotional Intelligence Test (SSEIT) to be of interest. It was developed by Dr. Nicola Schutte in 1998, and is described as "a method of measuring general Emotional Intelligence (EI), using four subscales: emotion perception, utilizing emotions, managing self-relevant emotions, and managing others' emotions."

Ask your sleep doctor about the PSQI or download the questionnaire at the pitt.edu website. You can easily find the EIS, or SSEIT questionnaire online. But stay focused here for now. Treat these tools as indicators, not gospel. Glean from them any insights that may help you focus on your sleep mastery.

Zzz-Tip: Accept the likelihood, as it has already been proven in others, that your emotional self-control directly impacts your sleep quality, and the lack of emotional self-control can impede your ability to sleep at night. Poor emotional self-control can lead to increased stress and anxiety, a precursor to, or a result of poor decision-making.

Program Your Mind with the Power of "I AM"

The power of positive, present-tense thought is indisputable. Our thoughts drive our behavior and our decision process, and create the very circumstances in which we find ourselves, in large part. However, we can take control of this process, and shape it for the better, when we utilize positive, present-tense thought.

In my clinical hypnosis practice, I teach the power of I AM to my clients as a core component of building self-confidence and courage to accept the self, and to face the world, by speaking truths to the subconscious mind. These two words, "*I AM,*" are the core of the truth that you declare to your mind that you are sleeping. The mind follows. There are various ways you can use the phrase, such as:

- I AM — two magic words by itself, revealed in the Bible, and explained for everyday living by R. J. Banks, Wayne Dyer, Joel Osteen, and Goddard Neville.
- I AM GOD — three magic words, as explained in Uell Stanley

Andersen's book *Three Magic Words: The Key to Power, Peace and Plenty*.

- I AM SLEEPING NOW — four magic words that invite sleep, in a matter-of-fact way.

The application of the I AM affirmation is infinite. These three affirmations mentioned above — along with many others which can incorporate the important phrase "I AM" — have an amazing compounding effect when you combine them, or when you "own them," and embrace them one at a time. The key is using self-hypnosis to program your mind accordingly.

We become what we think about, as I mentioned earlier in this book, and as referenced in the Bible. Where our attention goes, our energy flows. We have the power to choose, to program our mind to lead us in the direction we want to move. With courage enough, confidence enough, and determination enough, we can make progress and take control of our life. Right thoughts lead to right actions.

In James Allen's early 20th-century classic self-help book, *As a Man Thinketh*, he speaks of dreams and visions, and of taking action that leads us to the life we want to lead. Regarding vision and ideas, he says:

> In all human affairs there are efforts, and there are results, and the strength of the effort is the measure of the result. Chance is not. Gifts, powers, material, intellectual, and spiritual possessions are the fruits of effort; they are thoughts completed, objects accomplished, visions realized. The Vision that you glorify in your mind, the Ideal that you enthrone in your heart—this you will build your life by, this you will become.

Speaking of dreams, he writes:

> Dream lofty dreams, and as you dream, so shall you become. Your vision is the promise of what you shall one day be; your Ideal is the prophecy of what you shall at last unveil. The greatest achievement was at first and for a time a dream. The oak sleeps in the acorn; the bird waits in the egg;

and in the highest vision of the soul a waking angel stirs.
Dreams are the seedlings of realities.

As a Man Thinketh is a timeless book, by the way, and one well
worth reading. I've included a copy of it in the resource down-
loads at www.iamsleeping.com.

What's my point in all this, you ask?

I am confident the shift you seek, with the intention of inviting sleep back into your life, is already happening. What are you
dreaming about in your waking hours? In sleep, REM sleep specifically, your nighttime dreams may reveal insights. What actions are you taking during your waking hours that help your
dream of sleeping better come true?

By combining the power of autosuggestion (positive-inten-
tioned self-talk) with self-hypnosis, you create rapid reprogram-
ming of your mind, set by your intention. Learning to feed your
mind powerful, positive, present-tense thoughts in the conscious
state can be quite effective. You accelerate the progress and your
ultimate success when you speak directly to your subconscious
mind, using self-hypnosis. As Dr. Richard Nongard says, "Self-
hypnosis is so easy a child can do it. The journal *Pediatrics* reported that children who suffered from migraine headaches and
were taught self-hypnosis had a 63% reduction in both fre-
quency and severity and it was more effective than medication."
(Karen Olness, 1987)

Nongard also states:

> We act on what we believe, but unfortunately, much of
> what we believe about ourselves and our situations is
> simply false. Autosuggestion, developed by Émile Coué, is
> one of the easiest ways to practice self-hypnosis and has
> been used for more than 100 years. One of the best defini-
> tions for autosuggestion is a psychological technique re-
> lated to the placebo effect, developed by apothecary Émile
> Coué at the beginning of the 20th century. It is a form of
> self-induced suggestion in which individuals guide their
> own thoughts, feelings, or behavior. The technique is often
> used in self-hypnosis.

You have been introduced to Émile Coué already, in fact. He is best known for his famous autosuggestion, "Every day, in every way, I am getting better and better," paraphrased earlier. His work started a worldwide self-help movement in the early 1900s.

While Coué is credited with the discovery of autosuggestion in the modern era, the idea of feeding one's mind with healthy, positive thoughts goes back a long way. Shakespeare spoke using positive affirmations (e.g., the Bard's "To thine own self be true"), and St. Patrick and St. Augustine both professed the use of I AM in conscious programming. It was also espoused by the 4th-century Celts of Ireland, by the Roman Empire, and by the ancient Greeks like Aristotle, the Delphic Oracles of the Temple of Apollo, Pythagoras of Samos (who taught his Pythagorean disciples the principles of autosuggestion), and even as far back as Thales of Miletus (generally regarded as the very first philosopher in the Western tradition, and one of the Seven Sages of Greece in the 6th century B.C. — the same time period when Aesop lived and wrote his famous fables). Thales' "Know thyself" and "nothing too much" are two great examples. (Keep in mind, it was the citizens of Delphi, as wise philosophers they were, that tossed Aesop over a cliff to the sea, because he was smarter than them all!) Moving back up in time, to a slightly more recent history of affirmations, Benjamin Franklin, as published in his *Poor Richard's Almanack* in 1750, observed the great difficulty of knowing oneself, with: "There are three Things extreamly [sic] hard, Steel, a Diamond and to know one's self."

You knew this was coming, so let me ask: How well do you really know yourself? It's a lifelong relationship, this thing between you and yourself, but happiness requires your greater attention to this.

But let's keep this in the modern era for our purposes of helping you to use conscious affirmations and visualization to help you sleep!

As Émile Coué says in his book, *I Am Getting Better and Better: My Method*:

> Pythagoras and Aristotle taught auto-suggestion. We know,

indeed, that the whole human organism is governed by the nervous system, the center of which is the brain — the seat of thought. In other words, the brain, or mind, controls every cell, every organ, every function of the body. That being so, is it not clear that by means of thought we are the absolute masters of our physical organism and that, as the Ancients showed centuries ago, thought — or suggestion — can and does produce disease or cure it? Pythagoras taught the principle of auto-suggestion to his disciples. He wrote: "God the Father, deliver them from their sufferings, and show them what supernatural power is at their call."

Apply this Pythagorean practice, as he taught: When waking up, ask yourself, "How will I use today?" Before going to sleep, ask yourself, "What have I accomplished using this day?" One of his other thought-provoking sayings was, "The oldest, shortest words — *yes* and *no* — are those which require the most thought." Apply this! Say "yes" to committed changes for better sleep. Say "no" to the self-sabotage that has kept sleep away. Give thought to this.

Zzz-Tip: In all likelihood, autosuggestion probably goes right back to the beginning of language. Self-talk is not new, but we know it's powerful, both negatively and positively, so isn't it wiser to be in control? Although Coué's book was first published in 1923, long before modern medical science proved the benefits of autosuggestion, it is still a worthy reading adventure. You'll find it in the Resources section at www.iamsleepingnow.com.

Here we are, deep in this book, and I am about to state the obvious! *There is amazing mind-boggling power in our words.* As soon as we learn to speak, and even beforehand, when we are led by non-verbal cues, we begin to program ourselves using our self-talk. We are constantly programming ourselves with the words we use, spoken outwardly or inwardly. So, be ever vigilant in the words you choose to speak within or to others. Kindness and compassion, empathy, and sense of love are all important here.

Know that you can, with your words, program your thoughts and take your life in the direction you desire, and you have great influence in providing guidance to others. Choose good words, starting with "I AM." As author R. J. Banks says in his book, *The Power of I AM and the Law of Attraction*, "These two small words possess incredible, life-altering power, more than all others." The words "I AM" are yours and yours alone. No one else can say them for you. What follows these two simple words, says Banks, "will determine what type of life you have and will either, by the words you choose to use, bring success or failure in your life." Choose success, learn from failure. Use good self-talk. As Banks also says in his book, "When you say, 'I AM' and concentrate on positive things, you create positive experiences in your life." You know this to be true, I am certain.

Learn from the sages of the ages when it comes to autosuggestion and the power of I AM. It's found throughout ancient literature, including the Old Testament. Although this book is not a religious essay, as found in Exodus 3:11–15, the power of I AM is used by God when he appeared within the flames of a burning bush to instruct Moses. The passage is as follows:

> [11] But Moses said to God, "Who am I that I should go to Pharaoh and bring the Israelites out of Egypt?"
>
> [12] And God said, "I will be with you. And this will be the sign to you that it is I who have sent you: When you have brought the people out of Egypt, you will worship God on this mountain."
>
> [13] Moses said to God, "Suppose I go to the Israelites and say to them, 'The God of your fathers has sent me to you,' and they ask me, 'What is his name?' Then what shall I tell them?"
>
> [14] God said to Moses, "I AM WHO I AM. This is what you are to say to the Israelites: 'I AM has sent me to you.'"
>
> [15] God also said to Moses, "Say to the Israelites, 'The LORD, the God of your fathers—the God of Abraham, the God of Isaac and the God of Jacob—has sent me to you.'"

This all fits in with emotional self-control, visualizing the positive outcome you desire, and realizing that with a change in your thinking you can take back control of your emotions, and make better decisions in daily life. As a clinical hypnotist and coach, as a parent, and throughout my life as I faced my own challenges of confidence, esteem, and in even the tiniest of decisions, being mindfully aware of my I AMs has always guided me to the right place. It will for you as well — including preparing your mind for sleep with "I AM sleeping now"!

Your I AM affirmations must be present-tense, and positive in their formation. If I said, "I am going to go to sleep," well, that is in the future. Remember, the mind and body work closely together. The subconscious mind works in the present, not the past or future, albeit driven by intentions. When we consciously mold our beliefs by speaking directly to our subconscious, we can influence our destiny. Be aware that with better programming, you begin to make deep changes within yourself. And not only that, but amazingly, you seem to influence others as well, simply by your example. It's almost magical, and all for your highest and best.

Each new positive thought you adopt into your mind programming makes space for allowing what you do want in your life. Let me offer some suggestions here, as examples of positive affirmations that could apply to your life, including but not limited to your sleep self-programming, and in no particular order. Try saying them aloud and see which ones resonate:

- I am healthy and make healthy choices.
- I am safe and secure.
- I am guided by my higher source, my God.
- I am on a weight loss journey.
- I am thankful.
- I am brave, courageous, and strong.
- I love myself.
- I am enthusiastic and energetic.
- I revere and respect my sleep time.
- I am blessed with many gifts and talents.
- I am happy.
- I am in control of my emotions and behavior.
- I am calm, relaxed, and in control of my emotions.
- I am spiritual.
- I am in a healthy relationship with myself and with others.

- I am kind to myself and others.
- I am persistent in whatever I set out to accomplish.
- I am better and better every day.
- I am [your name], and I am alive.
- I am sorry.
- I am okay.
- I am grateful for my mind and body.
- I am aware of habits I should change in my pre-sleep routine.
- I am enough.
- I am ready for sleep.
- I am wholly and completely capable of falling and staying asleep.
- I am worthy and deserving of the sleep I seek now.
- I am sleeping now.

Well, that certainly was a long chapter.

Who ever thought so many words were needed to explain four simple words: *"I Am Sleeping Now."* You know at this point, that this is a journey that prepares you for sleep and for improving your awake state!

Next: Let's help you recharge during the day — even on those days when you arise refreshed and rejuvenated.

CHAPTER SIX

Recharge and Rejuvenate with a Hypnotic Power Nap!

"A day without a nap is like a cupcake without frosting."
—Terri Guillemets

I don't eat too many cupcakes these days but when I do, I have to have frosting. And just like with the cupcake, a day with a short power nap tastes just as sweet.

Is it true that those who nap during the day enjoy a better sex life and make more money, as some people have suggested? Not sure, but I am taking a snooze as soon as I complete this chapter!

In any case, why not modify "I Am Sleeping Now" to "I Am Napping Now" when a short power break is called for? Hmmm.

Remember nap time in kindergarten? Ah, it was so long ago. And so much fun, too. Those were the days. With all this talk about sleep in these pages, I thought that napping deserved its own place of reverence, since all signs — despite what you may initially think — lead to it being a solid contributor to the quality of your nighttime sleep. Leading experts, as you will see, endorse the short power nap (consisting of 10–30 minutes maximum), insisting that it brings a myriad of health benefits, and evidence seems to show that napping in this way does not interfere what-soever with nighttime sleep.

"You miss 100% of the naps you don't take."
—humorous take on a Wayne Gretzky quote

So, let's get you napping your way to success.

After all, napping is an established, culturally accepted practice across the globe. If you are a busy, Type-A personality who has often struggled to relax and enjoy the silence, this chapter may be particularly challenging. It's been my experience, however, that while those with this type of personality may typically view napping as a waste of time, after getting the hang of a short hypno-nap, they are hooked. They end up getting more done, with less angst, less stress, and a greater feeling of self-control over their destiny. You can, indeed, chart a new course in your life by adding a short power nap to your daily routine.

The Health Benefits of a Quick Power Nap

I call it hypnotic napping, and it's nothing new. It's simply your turn to start enjoying the benefit derived. A hypnotic power nap, which is 12 minutes maximum, offers a host of benefits, as you might imagine. Consider it if you find yourself with low energy right after the noon hour, or if you need that extra boost to round off your workday.

As verywellmind.com says:

> Sleep is cumulative; if you lose sleep one day, you feel it the next. If you miss adequate sleep several days in a row, you build up a 'sleep deficit', which impairs the following:
> - Reaction time
> - Judgment
> - Vision
> - Information processing
> - Short-term memory
> - Performance
> - Motivation
> - Vigilance
> - Patience

You might just be amazed at the positive effects of a short hypnotic power nap. You'll feel like, as they say, you "slept at a Holiday Inn Express," or like you just had a V8! My 12-minute rule is based on the fact that time distortion takes place in light hypnosis and you feel as if you were asleep for 30 minutes or so.

According to the Sleep Foundation:

> One significant factor responsible for the varied effects of naps is their length. Anytime we fall asleep, we begin to move through a series of sleep stages. Researchers found that five-minute naps are too short to move deep enough through sleep stages to produce a notable benefit. On the other hand, sleeping for 30 minutes or longer gives the body enough time to enter deep (slow wave) sleep. However, napping for too long or waking up from slow-wave sleep can leave you feeling groggy for up to an hour. This period of drowsiness is also called "sleep inertia."

> Given these considerations, the best nap length in most situations is one that is long enough to be refreshing but not so long that sleep inertia occurs. Naps lasting 10 to 20 minutes are considered the ideal length. They are sometimes referred to as "power naps" because they provide recovery benefits without leaving the napper feeling sleepy afterward.

The X-Factor in Business: The Power Nap Strategy

Hey, wouldn't you sometimes love to tell your boss to "go take a nap and let's talk about this later"? Of course you would, and perhaps you may have thought about saying it already.

But what if you were to tell your boss that *you* wanted to take a nap? What do you think they'd say? Well, believe it or not, he or she might just give you unexpected support! The truth of the matter is, sleep is becoming the new X-factor in business, and senior executives and business owners know the power of napping. In fact, the world's leading health and wellness experts agree; adult nap time is beneficial. The adage "you snooze you lose" suggests that sleep or napping is for the losers in life, but sleeping on the job — or, more precisely, *at* the job — is proving quite powerful, especially for that post-lunchtime push for the day. Short napping can help reduce stress and give you the necessary break your brain needs, making you sharper for the rest of the day. It may be time to rethink the 15-minute afternoon coffee break and take a short power nap instead! It's about taking a brief time out, so you don't burn out. Sleep and short power napping can impact the company's performance, service quality, morale, and even the bottom line.

When you embrace napping, you'll be joining the sages of the ages who made napping a part of their life. You'll also be joining, perhaps more importantly, the unsung heroes who keep the world running. The shift worker deprived of sleep, and the common man and woman who toil in their job to keep the rest of us safe and the economy moving forward. The fatigued over-the-road truck driver pulling off the highway to sleep.

Keep in mind there are two types of nappers — those who openly celebrate their nap time, and those who hide it (as a personal trade secret!). It is becoming more widely accepted and companies are encouraging napping in more and more cases. Talk to your boss about it, and if you are the boss, be open to the idea. Your employees will respond!

As discussed in *HuffPost*, Arianna Huffington, co-founder of *The Huffington Post*, had this to say on NBC's *Today* show: "Sleep makes us more productive, creative, less stressed and much healthier and happier. Even a 20-minute nap in the middle of the day can make a huge difference. I grew up thinking that if you work around the clock, you are going to be more effective, and I realize that is not true."

True confession! I take a short power nap almost every day at work when the opportunity exists, usually if I have a client cancellation or there's a gap. There is always plenty of work to be done, and it gets done more effectively and efficiently on the days when I can squeeze in a few daytime ZZZs. In this chapter, I will share my technique for a quick, rejuvenating self-hypnotic power nap.

Just as I seek to find the time to grab that daytime boost, I wonder if it is something you will add to your sleep mastery skills as well. Heck, step away from the internet for 20 minutes, put your phone down, and do your mind and body a favor. Your colleagues, co-workers, employees and customers (if you're a business owner), and family and friends will all appreciate you taking a short nap.

Combine a good night's sleep with a daily strategic power nap and, man, you are going places. What a one–two power punch to give you that career fast-track, or to simply make you feel good each day whether you be working, retired, or a student of any age!

The experts agree:
- Harvard University
- Johns Hopkins
- Mayo Clinic
- National Sleep Foundation
- National Institutes of Health
- Center for Disease Control
- Health.Gov
- American Psychological Association
- NASA

Let's face it, though: Despite the experts weighing in, napping is not culturally accepted in much of the Western hemisphere, is it? Well, what say you and I start to change that, one snoozing nap at a time!

By the way, investors and manufacturers of sleep products are aware of the growing interest in sleep. The whole world is getting less sleep on average, and you might even agree that sleeplessness is an ongoing and growing pandemic. As I mentioned earlier, the sleep product industry is estimated to be a $30B market annually, for the next several years.

It's both fascinating to observe and frustrating to see so much "expert" sleep advice coming from so-called sleep doctors, legitimate sleep doctors, mattress companies, technologists, supplement companies, etc., all trying to lead you to a product sale they claim will solve your sleep issues. The best sleep device you can ever own, you already have, as I have said, and it's between your ears. Unless you have a physical issue preventing sleep, mind–

body conditioning will do the trick — and napping only enhances your progress on this daily intention of waking up refreshed to enjoy the day!

Anyway, back to napping.

Sleep and short power napping can impact well-being overall. It's been researched and studied. A Japanese study, "The effects of a 20 min nap in the mid-afternoon on mood, performance and EEG activity," by Hayashi, Watanabe, and Hori, suggests that napping bolsters mood, and boosts professional and personal productivity. From the study: "The 20 min nap improved the subjective sleepiness, performance level and self-confidence of their task performance. The results suggest that a short 20 min nap in the mid-afternoon had positive effects upon the maintenance of the daytime vigilance level."

Another study published at the NIH, titled, "Good sleep, bad sleep! The role of daytime naps in healthy adults," by Dhand and Sohal, states:

> A nap during the afternoon restores wakefulness and promotes performance and learning. Several investigators have shown that napping for as short as 10 min improves performance. Naps of less than 30 min duration confer several benefits, whereas longer naps are associated with a loss of productivity and sleep inertia. Recent epidemiological studies indicate that frequent and longer naps may lead to adverse long-term health effects.
>
> A nap of less than 30-min duration during the day promotes wakefulness and enhances performance and learning ability. The benefits of napping could be best obtained by training the body and mind to awaken after a short nap.

ZZZ-TIP: Based on 13 years of experience speaking on the subject and in clinical work at my practice, hypnotic napping is the solution to managing your new habit of short power naps. The key is to avoid sleep inertia, which happens when you allow a nap to go on too long and fall into a deeper sleep. A hypnotic nap brings you into a light state that approximates sleep — but is not sleep at all. Brain waves slow, heart rate slows, body temperature drops, oxygen and blood flow increase as a result, and every cell in your body enjoys the rejuvenating experience. Heart–brain coherence creates calmness. The goal of hypnotic napping is to quickly teach the mind and body to relax, which this book is guiding you to learn. Using self-hypnosis to descend into your power nap simulates Stage 2 of the four stages of sleep, which is the place you want to be for the power nap — short, sweet, and restorative. If you limit your hypnotic power nap to about 10–12 minutes, you prevent your brain from falling to a deeper level.

Incidentally, during Stage 2 sleep, brain activity slows, for the most part, but bursts of rapid, rhythmic brain wave activity known as "sleep spindles" also occurs, that help us resist being woken up by external stimuli. They've also been found to be associated with the integration of new information into existing knowledge, which may help to explain those times when you doze for a moment and a creative idea or solution pops into your head!

Okay, apologies for that short scientific detour. Let's resume, shall we?

I should point out that very few sources, if any, even mention self-hypnosis as a power nap strategy. Business leaders are listening to sleep researchers, and they are embracing the importance of napping as a workforce health and performance advantage. While they may practice self-hypnosis, they may not feel comfortable revealing it, because, as I know from experience, people have preconceived notions about hypnosis — which highlights their lack of knowledge about the subject. People tend to dismiss what they do not understand, until they understand it. Make sense? Unfortunately, hypnosis is not widely understood except by those who have discovered its awesome power, including and far beyond our discussion on napping.

Of course, the proof is in the pudding and as you experiment with brief hypnotic naps, you'll find lots of ways to use it. It can be a short nap in the work setting, in the car (parked, and with the engine off, please!), at home on the deck, or maybe even at the beach. With skills mastery, you can give yourself a hypnotic suggestion literally anywhere. This book teaches enough about self-hypnosis for your success in sleep mastery, specifically. There are many books on the market today on the wider subject of self-hypnosis (and the benefits thereof), however. I recommend Dr. Richard Nongard's book, *The Self-Hypnosis Solution*. In fact, I give a copy of this book to every client of mine wanting to learn more. Of course there are many others, but Dr. Nongard's is written for modern times and is very easy to read.

The Self-Hypnotic Power Nap

As you know by this point in the book, hypnosis is an evidence-based, complementary, and often primary solution for aiding in goal progress, intentions, and, as in our case, for sleep! It holds true for napping as well. Since all hypnosis is self-hypnosis, that means that you are in charge and when your intention is a brief restorative nap, then only you can make it happen. No worries, though, it's pretty easy to learn, and practice leads to mastery!

I was first introduced to the idea of self-hypnosis while I was in the Navy, aboard a submarine. While in port each month, the boat received a substantial delivery of books for the ship's library. Most were snatched up immediately by the crew. I happened to get lucky, grabbing a book on hypnosis by Melvin Powers. I found his book, *A Practical Guide to Self-Hypnosis*, printed in 1961, quite fascinating. I used it for rapid sleep, as you never knew when you'd be awakened for who knows what, or when an alarm would sound. (The diving alarm, battle stations, reactor scram, or collision alarm, for instance, would frequently interrupt sleep —necessarily, I suppose!) I also used hypnosis to help my shipmates, as I was designated as the onboard alcohol and drug counselor. In that capacity, I only saw guys when the Commanding Officer would send them to me, when things got out of hand on shore. It was then that I really witnessed the power of suggestion firsthand, teaching my crewmates some effective self-suggestions to help throttle back on things.

Who knew that decades later, after a successful marketing

career, I would become a clinical hypnotist? The power of hypnotic suggestion was in the back of my mind the whole time, all those years ago and ever since. But I digress.

In your journey to master hypnotic napping, which can also aid you in jumpstarting your evening sleep routine, rest assured there are significant findings that provide the evidence that with relaxation techniques and hypnotic suggestions (given to the self), hypnotic napping is easy to experience and is more beneficial than trying to take a nap consciously, without using the hypnotic approach.

The NIH offers the results of another relevant study, "Using relaxation techniques to improve sleep during naps," conducted by a team of 12 researchers, as follows:

> The deepening of short naps with RT involving hypnosis might be a successful non-pharmacological way to extend sleep duration and to deepen sleep in occupational settings.

> Napping seems to be an efficient way to counteract sleep loss effects on health, as well as a means to sustain alertness during an otherwise sleepless period. In particular, short daytime naps of less than 30 min, going to stage 2 sleep, have been shown to have positive effects on daytime alertness and/or performance after a normal night of sleep in young and elderly individuals, and after a night of restricted sleep.

> Non-REM sleep 2 (N2) during daytime naps has a recuperative power on subjective alertness and cognitive performance, and self-confidence.

> Hypnotic suggestion, music, and progressive muscle relaxation techniques have also been found to improve objective and subjective sleep efficiency.

> Short daytime naps have been shown to be effective at counteracting negative outcomes related to sleep debt with positive effects on daytime sleepiness and performance after a normal or restricted night of sleep.

A short hypnotic power nap can also be inspirational and

reveal the answer to a problem you are trying to solve or a question you are pondering. When you start power napping you will join the likes of John D. Rockefeller, Thomas Edison, Leonardo da Vinci, Salvador Dali, Winston Churchill, and, I am sure, many of the sages of the ages who snuck in a short nap each day! In fact, as mentioned in the Art of Manliness blog, "Churchill felt that his naps helped him get twice as much done each day. Naps were so sacrosanct to Churchill that he kept a bed in the Houses of Parliament and believed that napping was the key to his success in leading the country through the Battle of Britain."

As Churchill is well known for saying, "Nature has not intended mankind to work from eight in the morning until midnight without that refreshment of blessed oblivion which, even if it only lasts twenty minutes, is sufficient to renew all the vital forces."

Thomas Edison, as the Art of Manliness blog continues:

> [W]as something of a self-hating napper. He liked to boast about how hard he worked, how he slept only three or four hours a night, and how he would sometimes work for 72 hours straight. But in truth the key to his spectacular productivity was something he was loath to mention and hid from others: daily napping. Once when his friend Henry Ford paid a visit to his lab, Edison's assistant stopped him from going into the inventor's office because Edison was snoozing. Ford said, "But I thought Edison didn't sleep very much." To which the assistant answered, "He doesn't sleep very much at all, he just naps a lot."

So, if great minds can master the art of quick (hypnotic) naps to get them through the day, you can as well! After all, you have the same great mind. Nap your way to success and happiness.

Yours truly uses power naps and brief visits to hypnagogia to find inspiration for both my writing and my consulting work. In working with clients, I have used the conscious/semi-hypnotic nap to provide support and guide them to a state where judgment fades, creativity steps forward, and where early-stage dreaming occurs.

How to Take a 10–12 Minute Self-Hypnotic Power Nap

Are you ready to go to the "edges of sleep" for a refreshing power boost? Here's a secret to hypnotic napping. The secret is to simply do it, and to limit your time to 12 minutes.

Why the time limit? The goal is to enter what is called the hypnagogic state — that place between awake and asleep, just below the beta brain wave state, into the alpha state (but no further). Consider it a deliberate flirting with sleep, allowing you to enjoy a brief encounter so you can enjoy the therapeutic and cognitive benefits without falling into a groggy state afterwards. There is a well-proven link between intuition and hypnagogic reverie, with thoughts and images occurring during the onset of sleep, which would not occur consciously.

Hypnagogia is a "borderline state" at the initial phase of sleep, a place of pleasant hypnotic hallucinations, or deep relaxation where visualization abilities are heightened. It is that purposeful feeling one experiences as they move *toward* sleep, but not going to sleep. Salvador Dali perfected the 30-second micro-nap for inspiration, and it is said that Leonardo da Vinci did the same, with the intent of sparking inspiration and experiencing, in a quick lucid dream state, a vision or image of relevance. In this state, it feels like experiencing the moment in a vague and dreamy way. Dali's 30-second naps did allow for this to be realized, although just barely, given their brief time frame. As such, I suggest the 10–12 minute approach, as I said, and entering the early stages of your journey toward sleep to that delicate border between stage one (N1) and stage two (N2), but halting any further depth into theta!

Hypnagogia is not a new concept. Historically, there is evidence in the writings of Aristotle, and of Syrian philosopher Iamblichus, Italian physician and mathematician Girolamo Cardano, and the Elizabethan herbalist Simon Forman, to name just a few. The term hypnagogic was originally coined in the mid-1880s by French scholar Alfred Maury to name the state of consciousness during the onset of sleep. Additionally, many authors have referenced the hypnagogic state. Edgar Allan Poe,

113

for example, wrote of the "fancies" he experienced "only when I am on the brink of sleep, with the consciousness that I am so." And Charles Dickens' *Oliver Twist* contains an elaborate descripttion of the hypnagogic state in the 34th chapter.

From Dickens' work:

> There is a kind of sleep that steals upon us sometimes, which, while it holds the body prisoner, does not free the mind from a sense of things about it, and enable it to ramble at its pleasure. So far as an overpowering heaviness, a prostration of strength, and an utter inability to control our thoughts or power of motion, can be called sleep, this is it; and yet, we have a consciousness of all that is going on about us, and, if we dream at such a time, words which are really spoken, or sounds which really exist at the moment, accommodate themselves with surprising readiness to our visions, until reality and imagination become so strangely blended that it is afterwards almost matter of impossibility to separate the two.

Mary Wollstonecraft Shelley reported that her classic tale, *Frankenstein; or, The Modern Prometheus*, came to her as a series of hypnagogic images the evening after her group of friends agreed to compete for the best original Gothic horror tale ever written. Inspired by a stormy vacation in 1816 at Lake Geneva, Switzerland with her soon-to-be husband, Percy Bysshe Shelley, and accompanied by her stepsister Claire and their friend Lord Byron, among others, at only 19 years of age, Mary Shelley penned this classic story. Trapped inside with poor weather, they entertained themselves with German ghost stories, and Lord Byron challenged the group to each write a ghost story of their own. Shelley wrote *Frankenstein*, inspired by images and ideas created in her light state of hypnosis!

I share these sideroad insights, as I call them, to offer confidence and inspiration. Now, imagine you, using the power-napping hypnagogic state to inspire your next great work!

Here's a quick, funny story about power napping. Imagine the in-port watch on a submarine moored along the pier. It's the midwatch, that seemingly endless period of time between midnight and 0600. Of course, sleeping on watch is a no-no, so this never really happened... *wink, wink*. Anyway, one creative shipmate, a non-smoker, decided to intermittently light up a cigarette while sitting on watch in the torpedo room. It was his ingenious way of getting in little micro-naps. Not wanting to get caught nodding by the ship's officer of the day on periodic rounds, he would let each cigarette burn down to his fingers, whereupon the last of its burning embers would wake him. Ouch! True story. He went through a pack a night, never actually smoking one.

As an alternative to my old shipmate's rather painful method, I suggest, instead, that you find a nice phone app such as MindBell (sometimes referred to as Buddha Bell). Set a soft gentle bell for 12 minutes. Or, find a similar ring tone for your phone's timer.

Okay, so as we've learned, hypnagogia is the place to power nap. Ah, but how do you get there?

This is how I do it, and how I teach my clients. Warning: This can become a very pleasant habit. You'll be a different person — more productive, more charismatic, happier. Remember, too, that during a short hypnotic power nap, you are not asleep. You are fully aware of your surroundings and always in complete control. Also, don't *try* to take a power nap, *take* a power nap. There is a difference.

Follow these steps to get you started. You may want to keep a pen and pad nearby, for when you emerge from this experience, a fountain of ideas may begin to flow. You want to be ready to capture them.

1. Set aside 15 minutes of undisturbed time. In an office set-ting, close your door with instructions not to be disturbed. Failing that luxury, go to your car during your lunch hour. Go park in the shade if possible. The idea is to find some safe solitude for your power ZZZs! At home, find a comfortable chair. A kitchen chair will do. Do not use your bed, do not lie down on the couch. No music. No TV. I often will do this at home on the back deck, or in the office, in my office chair. You can also do this on a trailside

boulder or log, or sitting at the beach! Anywhere you can be undisturbed for a bit.

2. Silence incoming calls on your phone, and look toward the next 12 minutes as a well-deserved timeout for your boost or rejuvenation. Sit comfortably.

3. Set your timer for 12 minutes. Do not start it just yet.

4. Take a nice deep breath, in through your nose. Hold it gently, and exhale through your mouth. Do this for a couple of minutes as you anticipate the pleasure of emerging from your nap, feeling recharged and refreshed.

5. Now, start your timer.

6. Allow your eyes to close as you take a nice, deep, cleansing breath and you say to yourself, "*I feel calm, I feel relaxed, I feel in control*"... and realize you are taking control of your mind and body in this moment, and as this happens, you begin to relax both physically and mentally.

7. Allow your eyes to close gently. Your eyelids are the easiest muscles to relax — an excellent mind–body connection, driven by your intention to nap! Focus on your breath, and your awareness that you are, indeed, relaxing quickly. Relax your arms, pretend if you must, and just imagine them so loose and limp, as if they were like a wet dishrag or a rag doll. Loose and limp. Heavy on the armrest or in your lap, or perhaps feeling light and floaty. Your choice.

8. Now, slowly count down, from seven down to zero, taking a slow relaxing breath as you do so. Nice breath in... and exhale... *Seven... six, relaxing away any stress and tension, and five... allowing your attention to stay focused on your breathing... four... relaxing deeper down now... that's right... letting all remaining stress melt away like the melting wax on a burning candle... three... two... as you might begin to notice... a color appears... no specific meaning... and if no color appears... so what... it may at a future time... just let it, when it does... no efforts... and one... deeply relaxed, yet*

away of your surroundings... without focusing on anything except the moment.

9. Allow whatever images or experiences to be revealed, without judgment.

10. Continue to say to yourself, *"I am calm, I am relaxed, I am in control of my thoughts and emotions."*

11. Do not try to accomplish anything specific. This is not about entering hypnosis to feed your mind a specific autosuggestion. Not yet anyway!

12. When the bell dings, take a deep breath, open your eyes, and sit in the stillness for a moment. Do not allow yourself to go back into the hypnagogic state, as tempting as it may feel. Emerge and go about your day.

13. After a couple of weeks of this practice, you can do some advanced power napping by adding one specific suggestion to aid you in being centered emotionally, and in all respects. Check the resource section of www.iamsleepingnow.com.

As Andreas Mavromatis explains in his 1987 book *Hypnagogia: The Unique State of Consciousness Between Wakefulness and Sleep*, "Thought processes on the edge of sleep tend to differ radically from those of ordinary wakefulness. For example, something that you agreed with within a state of hypnagogia may seem completely ridiculous to you in an awake state." Additionally, a 2001 study by Harvard psychologist Deirdre Barrett found that, while problems can also be solved in full-blown dreams from later stages of sleep, hypnagogia was especially likely to solve problems which benefit from hallucinatory images being critically examined while still before the eyes.

You can use the power nap to rejuvenate and recharge, to open your mind and invite new ideas and images into your realm, and even to have a brief conversation with God, if you are so inclined. When you are in prayerful thought, you are in a light hypnagogic state. Try it.

So, to sum it up... wherever and whenever you can, take a 12-

minute hypnotic power nap! It will change your life over time, and it is good practice for falling asleep as well!

CHAPTER SEVEN

Anchors Away!

"Why should the actions of the imagination not be as real as those of perception?"
—Gaston Bachelard, Philosopher

O h, the sailor in me would love to be using the title of this chapter in strictly the nautical sense only! But, alas, the anchors I refer to are those that buoy the mind and body, enabling action and a self-conditioned response, and driven by our very own intentions.

For those not nautically inclined, the phrase is properly spelled "anchors aweigh," and means the anchors are no longer rested on the bottom of the sea and that the ship is officially underway, on its charted course. And your ship, by the way, the sleek and mighty S.S. *Sleep Easy*, should be well underway by this point!

In nautical terms, an anchor stabilizes a ship to a solid reference point and, as I write this, it stirs a memory of our submarine anchored in Hong Kong's Victoria Harbour, a busy world port, where we were moored to an imaginary point on a harbor chart, right off the sea lane, secured by the resting anchor at the bottom of the harbor. I want to present another sort of anchor, however — one that buoys you to the relaxed state that can bring sleep right to your door. In mind/body conditioning, the anchor metaphor is perfect as it creates a connection to a particular psychological reference state, enabling you to stabilize and control yourself in any given situation.

This chapter is about using an anchor — be it a word, gesture, thought, image, or color — to associate or connect to an emotional state or feeling. For example, ever see a person squeeze their fist, pump their arm, and say "yes!" when they were extremely happy in the moment?

Imagine for a moment that you are lying comfortably in a cozy bed. Pretend for a moment that you can gently rise up and out of your body and float to the corner of the room and observe yourself sleeping. Now, as you watch that scene, enjoying the image of you sleeping soundly, begin to focus in on the peaceful feeling that comes with knowing that you can, indeed, sleep like that again — consistently — and that the sleep you are inviting back into your life is finding its way back to you. Take a deep breath, smile, and float right back into that image of yourself sleeping peacefully in the bed.

Connect the feeling of knowing that peaceful, restful sleep is within reach. Now, in what is referred to as the peak of this resource state, connect it to a word, a touch, a gesture — anything that allows you to recall the state when you want it to appear! Anchor it; associate the thought and feeling with triggers that you can install.

An Easy-to-Use Tool for Self-Empowerment

When working with clients, I always teach self-hypnosis techniques, some of which you are learning in this book. I teach the power of autosuggestion, mental rehearsal, visualization, and such. The topic of anchoring is always part of the self-empowerment skills-building process, too.

Anchoring is a tool in mind/body conditioning that can be helpful in infinite ways, including having more confidence in a situation, taking your enthusiasm to new heights as needed, or feeling calmer, relaxed, and more in control of thoughts and emotions. Any situation. It refers to the mental and physical process of associating an internal response or feeling with an external or internal trigger that can quickly call up a response, as needed, in any situation. It is a powerful tool to help you change your resource state on command, using your installed associative trigger. An anchor carries an emotional charge — call it a spark — that can instantly change a mind state.

Anchoring is in our everyday life as well and it's called conditioned response. This response, whether installed by others in your environment or by your own actions, can be accessed any time, and even covertly when the situation dictates, such as when walking up to the podium to make a speech, for example. Setting personal anchors will be integral as you take back control of your sleep!

Keep in mind that an anchor can elicit a positive or a negative response.

Entering your resource state on demand, like at the push of a button, is entirely possible and, in fact, is a strategy used by executives, athletes, and people from all walks of life. Anchors are used in marketing as a very powerful association with a brand experience.

Here are a few examples of anchoring in everyday life:

- The doorbell rings, a siren sounds, or the phone rings. The sound triggers your response to take appropriate action. That's an anchor.
- The smell of a favorite Sunday dinner may bring you back to a memory of a happy time in your childhood, at Grandma's house or a family gathering you hosted, with all of your loved ones at the table.
- The sound of a dentist's drill can conjure up fear of pain. The good news is that this negative anchor can be collapsed and replaced with a positive association!
- A baby crying for attention. It's an ear-piercing sound, a natural condition/response stimulus, intended to bring a parent's focus to their baby's needs, be it sleep, a diaper change, or a fresh bottle.
- The smell of suntan lotion may bring up a memory of a favorite vacation or a visit to the beach.
- A song on the radio may trigger any of a wide range of

emotions. Advertisers use music to tap into your subconscious mind and access your anchors!

- A traffic light turns yellow or red and you prepare to stop your vehicle, or brake lights in the car ahead of you cue you to stop or slow down. Anchor.

- A salesperson walking into the prospect's office to win the opportunity can anchor their confidence and also visualize the customer accepting the proposal — anchoring and future pacing the outcome, all with a single word, a touch of the ear, or whatever they 'installed' as their personal trigger.

- A golfer struggling to let go of a disappointing previous swing so the poor performance off the tee does not adversely affect their next shot or ruin their entire game. Sliding the club into the bag, or handing it to a caddy, can be an anchor to let go of the shot. An internal anchor can quickly reinstall their confidence, and the focus pivots and turns to the current shot.

- On a personal note, from my days in the submarine force, anchors were used to keep things on an even keel, so to speak. The diving alarm caused a certain automatic response, for instance, as did the battle stations alarm.

In my clinical hypnosis practice, I have helped clients to anchor themselves to take back control in a wide range of situations. I've also helped them to uninstall negative anchors that were impacting their lives adversely and holding them back. (Contact me if you need help in this area!) I've also taught people from all walks of life to use anchoring as a strategic tool to make an important change. Anchoring is a very simple way to help you change a resource state, as I mentioned, to help you reach within to find that inner resource you need in the present moment. It is such a cool tool for your personal state control, and it will have a tremendously positive impact on your entire life as you master this new skill.

Here are a few client success stories, where anchoring that

was created in hypnosis caused the shifts they were seeking, allowing them to re-access their resource state:

- A high school girl wanting to excel in her dance competitions anchored her performance confidence and reframed herself by taking a relaxing deep breath (an anchor) and saying to herself, "story time," and tugging on her left ear. She realized how easily she could get lost in telling her story on stage, using her body to communicate.

- A marketing executive needed to uninstall a negative anchor that arose every time he saw his father's number on the caller ID of his phone. Anchoring became a part of his clinical therapy work to create a new positive, welcoming feeling when his father would call.

- A church singer with exceptional skills feared a certain note in a requested song and at the altar always anticipated a problem. Anchoring her past success led her to easily ignore the feared musical note as it arrived in the song, and she gained confidence over the issue.

- A room of 250 people, all who were in attendance to learn how to lower their anxiety and stress and learn to fall asleep easier. I helped them install an anchor that easily helped them access a helpful resource state.

- A six-year-old boy who had difficulty focusing in the classroom and paying attention to the teacher. His behavior was troublesome in class, and he was not going to be allowed to stay enrolled in his school. By teaching him to anchor his desire to please his teacher, a simple hand-squeeze under his desk brought about his calm focus. Easy.

- I've even learned to put my fiancée's two cockatiels into a mesmerized state when it's time for them to return to their cages for the evening! In actuality, it's just anchoring. I'll continually distract one of them as he sits on my arm and I walk toward the cage. He likes being called a "pretty bird" by me. He has anchored this little ritual with his (cooperative) journey to his cage. Easy. For the other bird, I close one door to the cage, and leave the other half-open. When she sees it, she walks right in, knowing it's sleep time. Funny, but true.

Now, imagine how it is going to be, as you go from feelings of anxiousness about sleep onset to a feeling of complete control and confidence as you anchor yourself to such a relaxed mental and physical state that sleep comes easily (and using your anchor, as well, to fall back asleep should you awaken during the night). The magic is happening already, isn't it?

Here are five easy steps to help you install an anchor:

1. First, determine how you want to feel in a particular situation. It could be having more motivation, summoning up more energy from within, having more confidence, being more focused, or simply being more relaxed and less stressed in the moment. Decide on that super feeling you want to enjoy.

2. Recall a time, a memory, of when you felt that state before — a strong recollection of that experience. It could be a long-ago memory, or something more recent. As you breathe and relax, something will emerge. It could even be a time when you recall awakening refreshed and ready for the day! Maybe on vacation. If you cannot recall a time, use your wonderful imagination to pretend you can!

3. Next, decide how you want to best anchor it in your mind. Choose a word, or a gesture — such as a light fist-clenching and pump of the forearm, or, what I often suggest, touching your index finger and thumb together making a circle.

4. Install the anchor. Connect with that recalled memory. Be there, with that memory, and feel now like you felt when it occurred. Create a vivid experience in your mind as you connect to it. Your mind has stored that feeling and you can associate and recall it. Begin to re-experience the memory as if it were happening now. As the intensity of that feeling comes right back to you, *activate your chosen anchor* and install this mind/body conditioned response! Let that imagery and feeling come over you — sharper, in greater

intensity and focus, in full color. Take a relaxing breath and apply the anchor you've chosen. Again, I suggest touching your thumb and finger as your anchoring trigger.

5. You can practice and test the anchor by repeating it, without skepticism or resistance. This will strengthen the anchor's influence as you bring about the desired anchored resource state. Simply break the state intentionally. Use the anchor to bring the desired state right back!

Let's create an anchor that will become useful later in this book, and, more importantly, in your sleep routine as you prepare for sleep! You'll find it helpful throughout life in a variety of different situations, but right now we are focused on helping you to easily and quickly fall and stay asleep.

Anchoring for Any Desired State – Including Falling Asleep Fast

1. Take a few deep, slow, relaxing breaths. In through your nose… and out through your mouth.
2. Imagine that state you desire. Let's use "relaxed, calm, and in emotional control."
3. Now, touch your thumb and finger together as you intensify this feeling of relaxation and imagine yourself in complete control of your emotions. Tap gently, or rub, as if imagining a grain of sand between your fingertips.
4. Connect with how it feels to relax deeply… continue to breathe and allow yourself to relax more and more.
5. Tap again.
6. Repeat steps 4 and 5 again.
7. Enjoy this feeling and practice using this anchor throughout your day.
8. Now, use it each night as you prepare for hopping into bed for a good night's sleep.
9. More on this later. Use steps 1–7 to anchor any desired state.

Now, as Dr. Richard Nongard teaches in his Subliminal Science program on sleep, imagine for a moment "as your head hits the pillow, anchor the feel of your head touching the pillow as a signal that the ritual of sleep is about to begin." Your pillow can be your empowering, sleep-inviting anchor that enables you to embrace sleep as you practice your I AM SLEEPING NOW mastery skills.

Imagine you creating and installing stacked anchors as your sleep time approaches, letting the clock be an anchor to begin shifting toward a sleep routine.

- 2–3 hours before bed, you look at the clock, your appetite fades, and you enjoy a glass of water or a cup of green tea. This is a natural way to prepare your mind for sleep onset.
- See yourself logging off your email or the internet at least one hour before bed.
- Imagine you shifting to your pre-sleep routine 30 minutes before bed.
- Now imagine, 30 minutes prior to climbing into bed, that you take a few nice relaxing breaths, which will anchor your mind and body to your desired pre-sleep state of peace and harmony within.

As you will learn in Chapter Nine, when we discuss sleep rituals and routines in more detail, you'll begin to create new associations and triggers that help you jumpstart the pre-sleep relaxation that brings calmness and soothes the reticular activating system.

Our imagination allows us to create what we want in our minds, as I have been explaining, and with the courage, confidence, and a little commitment to the intention that is set, we take deliberate action toward the goal. Let's lightly touch on some key concepts that apply to those four magical words "*I Am Sleeping Now.*"

Yes. Let's set ourselves up for progress and success by understanding some of the phenomenal tools that help trigger our ability to easily fall asleep. Before we do, however, you do know the most important tool for aiding you in falling asleep when the time is appropriate, right? Simply decide to allow sleep to come to you and simply give yourself permission to go to sleep now. (Well, when I say "now," I don't mean it in the *literal* sense, of course. Keep reading, please. Although I am on a mission to help you sleep, I hope it's not my writing that is doing it for you!)

In the journey toward finding the comforting sleep that you seek, you'll discover each of these strategies combine to create a powerful set of tools, customizable by your own imagination. Each of these methods can help you anchor feelings from past successes right to the present moment, and to the outcome you desire. Recall the memory and the feeling. Connect with it in the present moment. Future pace yourself to the outcome as if it is already achieved in your mind. Anchor it. Install it. Repeat the process.

Zzz-TIP: You'll find more resources for positive anchoring techniques, as well as collapsing negative anchors, when you go to www.iamsleepingnow.com. Among the supporting techniques you'll find there include more on visualization, mental rehearsal, emotional freedom, and Dr. Richard Nongard's 3-2-1 anti-anxiety hug.

You can do that later, but for now, let's stay on course here as we end the chapter on a nautical note, just as we started it.

Anchors aweigh! Stay the course for true north. Imagine you, with your self-empowering anchors safely aboard — tested and ready for the high seas called life — able to better steer the S.S. *Sleep Easy*!

CHAPTER EIGHT

Clearing Obstacles Encountered on Your Sleep Journey

"The power of determination will make you unstoppable."
—The Honourable Jean J. Charest, Queen's Privy Council for Canada

This journey toward enjoying sleep once again is simply a part of your *unbeatable spirit*. You have the power to do anything you put your mind to do, and this is just the next focal point along the way. Clearing obstacles on our path to peace, happiness, and success creates breakthroughs — when you are willing to address such obstacles. But as a professional hypnotist, I know that this is a constant effort on the battlefield called our mind, or, to use a less contentious metaphor, on this journey called life, as we try our best to live our core values and purpose. As we travel through each day, we need to develop effective mental strategies for eliminating the obstacles.

The idea here, whether we're talking about sleep skill mastery or mastering any other aspect of our life, or simply wanting to maintain a sense of calm in our daily life, is to disempower any obstacle standing in our way. Rest assured that, as you might expect, there are many easy and powerful hypnotic techniques that will help you zap the obstacles away! The goal when you encounter any obstacle that impedes you is to, with courage and confidence, see yourself going above it, under it, around it, or right through it, unfazed — because you are unstoppable. In fact, as you progress through this book, and take in what resonates for your personal action plan, you begin to realize:

There is a new you beginning to emerge... connected to that true you found deep down inside... the person you are... as you say "I AM"... and begin to know... that peace comes naturally to you... as you live authentically... hypnotically... connecting your whole soul to the universe... living your full potential... mind... spirit... body... heart... and you acknowledge to yourself that no person, place, images, memories, words, thoughts from the past... the present... or into the future... can stop you from making your dreams become your reality... You are brave... courageous... and strong. You are unstoppable.

Zzz-Tip: Memorize the above autosuggestion. Write it out on an index card. Enter a state of light self-hypnosis and read it once a day for a week, as part of your journey toward welcoming sleep back into your life, and for more fully living each day!

The first step is awareness of the obstacles so that you can lighten your burden, and face any resistance, excuses, or what I call "creative avoidance" behaviors and habits that you have developed for that self-sabotage you've fostered.

- What is it, really, that is blocking you from sleeping well again?
- Are you allowing resistance to hold you back from doing what your wise mind knows you should be doing to invite sleep back into your life?
- Are you ready to stop chasing sleep, and start blasting away at the mental obstacles that have held you back?

You are adopting — or you can decide right now to do so — an unbeatable determination to return to the days of normal, organic, holistic sleep.

There is a song from 1983 called "Break My Stride" (written by Gregory Prestopino and Matthew Wilder, performed by Wilder, and covered by Love Cannon, Blue Lagoon, and Max-A-Million, along with a host of others). It was very popular at the time, and is relevant here in that the theme of the song is to not let anything or anybody slow or hold you down! Check out the song. You might find it inspirational in those moments where you start to notice fear, uncertainty, and doubt creeping in. You've got to "keep on movin'" — as the song tells us!

You have the power to clear or let go of the things that eat at you or otherwise impede your progress. Know that you are in the process of taking back control, and in choosing to be courageous, brave, and strong, you are freeing yourself to mindfully move toward conquering all that may be or once interfered with your sleep.

I am always amazed when I witness a client's revelation during our work together. In all my years in practice, it's exciting to see the client make progress simply by acknowledging the obstacles or tangents that can impede their journey to what it is they seek for themselves. You see, every client, at least as I have come to appreciate, brings with them the answer, or a clue to the answer, for the clinical hypnotist to use in forming what seem to be magical hypnotic suggestions. It's true for you, too, as you proceed on this journey to master your sleeping skills once again. In hypnosis, however lightly experienced, we can access that vast and wise resource within us that we refer to as our subconscious mind. This journey of yours is helping you do just that — to more easily access your wise mind.

We all encounter obstacles along our path, our journey in life. It's how we choose to address them, or not, that makes a difference. This welcoming path is a healing path, and this work you are doing right now is both transformative and healing — emotionally, physically, and mentally. For, as you know, sleeping well leads to living well, and this leads to a better connection with family, friends, co-workers, strangers you encounter, and also with God, who lies within you and in everyone you meet.

Keep in mind your triumphant victory over your sleeplessness. It's happening, and vigilance over the potential obstacles is key.

One of the biggest obstacles impeding success is resistance, also known as "self-sabotage." In his book *The War of Art* and in his follow-up book *Do the Work*, author Steven Pressfield talks about that ever-present nemesis — resistance — that pops up to sabotage us. Be aware of resistance and the negative self-talk it creates. Be courageous and do what you've put your mind to doing! Believe in yourself and hold yourself accountable.

You are overcoming resistance in this sleep mastery skills process. Resist resistance! Keep on going!

In my practice, I always use the metaphor of "The Welcoming Path," something I have developed along the way as an analogy for the journey of life. I will use it when I speak with clients about the choices they have — of walking life backwards, always living and looking back down the timeline of their past and never allowing themselves to live in the present, or, how they can pivot and face their present reality and choose to live hypnotically. The path, as I explain and suggest in hypnosis, connotes a certain sense of calmness and relief, I suppose. Clients connect with the metaphor and find a sense of peace within as they choose the right path for themselves, moving forward. You can do this, too.

For me, the notion of a peaceful, welcoming path first came to mind while reading *The Miracle of Mindfulness* by author Thich Nhat Hahn, a Buddhist monk, as he wrote from exile in Paris to his brother in Vietnam. Mindfully walking a meditative path, whether in the literal sense, or in the magical mind using mental rehearsal and visualization, is a healing experience that gives comfort and hope. I hope you will embrace it, both for yourself and for others!

A brief definition of mindfulness is perhaps appropriate here. Quite simply, as defined by Jon Kabat-Zinn, mindfulness is essentially paying attention on purpose with greater awareness and without judgment.

Further, as *Greater Good Magazine* explains, from their article at berkeley.edu:

> Mindfulness means maintaining a moment-by-moment awareness of our thoughts, feelings, bodily sensations, and surrounding environment, through a gentle, nurturing lens.
>
> Mindfulness also involves acceptance, meaning that we pay attention to our thoughts and feelings without judging them

— without believing, for instance, that there is a "right" or "wrong" way to think or feel in each moment. When we practice mindfulness, our thoughts tune into what we are sensing in the present moment rather than rehashing the past or imagining the future.

Though it has its roots in Buddhist meditation, a secular practice of mindfulness has entered the American mainstream in recent years, in part through the work of Jon Kabat-Zinn and his Mindfulness-Based Stress Reduction (MBSR) program, which he launched at the University of Massachusetts Medical School in 1979. Since that time, thousands of studies have documented the physical and mental health benefits of mindfulness in general and MBSR in particular, inspiring countless programs to adapt the MBSR model for schools, prisons, hospitals, veterans' centers, and beyond.

My own two cents on mindfulness?

Mindfulness is not a new concept. Long before the mindfulness movement of the 1980s and the explosion of mindfulness gurus on the internet today, mindfulness was being cultivated by the great philosophers of past centuries. Greek and Roman Stoic philosophers Epictetus, Seneca the Younger, and Marcus Aurelius have much to say on the subject, as they were teaching a way of living our daily lives. And others preceded them!

Walk your own mindfulness path as you tackle this challenge of sleeplessness. Look into the popular mindfulness books by Kabat-Zinn, Michael Yapko, and even Viktor Frankl's book *Man's Search for Meaning*, which is essentially a meditation on what the gruesome experience of Auschwitz taught him about the primary purpose of life (i.e., the quest for meaning). For Frankl, meaning came from three possible sources — purposeful work, love, and courage in the face of difficulty. What say you? Does this factor into your life as well?

In the book *The Miracle of Mindfulness*, mentioned just earlier, Thich Nhat Hahn offers several metaphors for present moment living. My two favorites are, "When it's time to wash the dishes, wash the dishes," and, "Chop wood, carry water." Both may be self-explanatory, but I'll briefly elaborate here.

In the first, he means that when it is your turn to do the dishes, embrace it without complaint and bring your best effort to the task. Focus on each dish and, with gratitude, mindfully be in the present moment and feel appreciative of the opportunity. In the second, as with washing the dishes, when it is your turn to do anything, any task, when that moment arrives, do it graciously, with a smile, and welcome the opportunity.

Now, back to the Welcoming Path!

In the office I will ask my client to envision a path, something they can see themselves walking on, enjoying a walking meditation in the right direction, whatever that means to them in the moment. The obstacles and opportunities along the way will present a chance for their growth mindset to develop as they, with an open mind, are able to see self-learnings along the way. I will often say:

Isn't it nice to know, finally, you are taking even the smallest of steps along this right path at this moment in your life? I can only imagine that your journey has taken you on other paths... and aren't we all on a journey back, anyway? A journey from the time of our birth, back to our creator... the human life so fragile... and dependent on the loving care of others until and sometimes far after we reach adulthood... and yet that child within us is always alive yet somehow dormant at times, for whatever reason... As you walk this path, imagine you are carrying a rucksack full of stones... and as you relax with every healing breath... you reach in and toss aside one stone... feeling what it feels like to walk a little lighter... more erect... feeling in more control and feeling more peace within you with each stone you cast aside... Let those stones be your letting go of whatever is holding you back... journey on, be it throughout your daily living, or as you journey toward sleep mastery!

I offer those words as a nice preamble as it sets the stage for introducing a variety of things along the welcoming path as they take bold, courageous, deliberate steps forward, just like the Tortoise in the Aesop's fable mentioned in an earlier chapter.

All of the above pertains to you as you tackle your sleep challenges!

As an example of a success story, Jeff was a client of mine who struggled to fall asleep. Yes, he consulted "Doctor Google" for his diagnosis, and the various groups of commiseraters on social media offered all kinds of concoctions and secret remedies. When he came to see me, his intention was to sleep better and get more sleep each night, and to do so without medications. He was embarrassed by the money he had spent previously on costly devices, pillows, and mattresses that offered the promise of deep sleep (but which hadn't delivered).

After Jeff made the positive decision to face what was keeping him awake and unable to fall asleep, I was then able to help him condition his mind, using the techniques presented in this book toward that end. Prior to our work, he viewed sleep as an annoying necessity. He had many demands on him stemming from his job, his family responsibilities, and his own personal goals. He was also a person who could not sit still.

We worked on the emotional issues affecting his life and used self-hypnosis skill-building and techniques that helped him to garner the courage to face what was ailing him. What he felt was deep regret and guilt, and he and I worked to put that in the right perspective so that he could sleep well once again. I would like to share one particular technique that worked for Jeff, and which may help you as well.

The Snow Globe Induction

Years ago, I created a self-hypnosis exercise that anyone can use along their journey toward becoming their best self. I call it the "Snow Globe" induction and deepener, designed to be an easy-to-use tool for reframing — to experience or see life differently.

Sometimes it is difficult to see things from a different perspective. Sometimes our perception causes an incomplete picture to be formed and, with cloudy thinking, we begin to think certain thoughts, feel certain ways, and act in certain ways based on what we perceive. With that in mind, the following exercise may help you to pause and reflect on things going on in your life that could be negatively impacting your ability to fall and stay asleep and wake up refreshed. Use this Snow Globe induction to help yourself bring forward any observations, as it relates to what might be in the way of progress, or to review or reflect on decisions that need to be made. Keep your intention in mind as you ponder this. Your subconscious mind is observing, too.

So without further ado, here is a short version of the Snow Globe induction, taken from my book, *The Magic of Aesop*:

Imagine holding a snow globe in your hand... shake it up and imagine seeing all the flakes begin to settle as you place the snow globe on the table in front of you... I wonder whether you can experience that scene in this moment... and as the flakes do begin to settle... take a couple of deep relaxing breaths... invite relaxation in... and as you watch the flakes settle... and you begin to notice how deep and relaxed your breathing has become... I wonder if you begin to feel a shift inside... a person does once in a while and it may be true for you as well... as the flakes settle, let that be a metaphor for your mind... your brain waves settling into a nice light hypnotic feeling of inner peace and tranquility... Imagine the snow globe along a path... the very path you are walking in life now... and walking around it... seeing what you are trying to see... that you can only see when the flakes settle... I wonder what you see... for in the center is YOU... and your life... see it from different angles... quietly observe... mindfully... let the center now become the very issue you may be struggling with to resolve... and just see it... from all sides... being open to see it from all angles... NOW... imagine walking right up to the door on the side of this magical snow globe... Open it and walk in... close it behind you now... and just raise your hand so I know you are there... Now... slowly and gently, without disturbing the settled flakes... walk to the center and find the nice comfortable swivel chair... sit... get comfortable... and begin to gaze outward... as you find that with enhanced clarity you begin to see what you need to see... obstacles... successes... tasks to focus on as you contemplate your intentions... and what is calling for your attention now... so now I am going to just be silent for a moment as you swivel and look around... out at what you see... and see if there is more to see... or feel... or touch... or smell... or any of your multisensory sensations... and now... begin to simply walk out of the snow globe... recharged... rejuvenated... resilient and refocused... as you step back onto the welcoming path... feeling great... at peace in knowing what you know is all you need to know now... all else reveals itself as you take small trusting steps each day... in fact... knowing that every day in every way you are better and better.

Feelings, Nothing but Feelings... and Desires!

Let's shift gears slightly as we stay with feelings, and your intention to sleep better. In the end, it is all about feelings and desires, right? Even if the desire is to have no desires (which is a subject for another day).

Emotional intelligence and self-control are the keys as you begin setting sail toward a new destiny as a person who has mastered sleep. Lao Tzu, the ancient Chinese philosopher, put it well: "Heed your thoughts; they become your words. Heed your words; they become your actions. Heed your actions; they become your habits. Heed your habits, they become your character. Heed your character, it becomes your destiny."

We become what we think about, and when we focus on self-mastery, self-accountability, and taking back control of our daily life in a greater way, then sleep will come back to you more naturally.

Lao Tzu, author of the influential *Tao Te Ching*, lived roughly the same time as Aesop, by the way, the two of them being contemporaries or near contemporaries. Interestingly, scholars have noticed distinct similarities between many of the morals of Aesop's Fables and the lessons found in the *Tao Te Ching*, despite the two authors being separated by thousands of miles! Over the centuries, from then and earlier to now, other cultures have handed down wisdom in the form of short stories and parables also. No accident, I suppose, that Jesus told many parables to the flock as well.

Remember that our thoughts lead to beliefs and feelings,

which in turn lead to actions and new behaviors (as Lao Tzu indicated in the aforementioned quote). Most of the time, this occurs automatically, triggered by our subconscious programming over the course of our life. We *can*, on occasion, take control of this process, however. Driven by our intentions, we can explore our behaviors and consciously involve ourselves in creating new neural network connections that cause the shift we seek!

In my work as change agent and facilitator on my clients' journey, helping them find the inner empowerment they need to make progress, I know that *no change can take place until change takes place.* In other words, the client needs to want the change and be willing to make change happen incrementally or all at once. As with my clients, you need to feel the feeling of the change already happening or having taken place!

Let's Let the Stoics Weigh In!

Briefly, since we've already mentioned a moment ago about the interesting similarities between the morals of Aesop's fables to the work of others, allow me to make note of Stoic philosopher Epictetus once again. His teachings were written down and compiled by his pupil, Arrian, in both *Enchiridion* and *Discourses*. In them, Epictetus is credited with these familiar, seemingly Aesopian, fable-like sayings:

- *"Men are disturbed not by things, but by the view which they take of them."*
- *"We have two ears and one mouth so that we can listen twice as much as we speak."*
- *"It's not what happens to you, but how you react to it that matters."*
- *"No man is free who is not master of himself."*
- *"There is only one way to happiness and that is to cease worrying about things which are beyond the power of our will."*
- *"First say to yourself what you would be; and then do what you have to do."*
- *"Only the educated are free."*

- *"Wealth consists not in having great possessions, but in having few wants."*
- *"It is impossible for a man to learn what he thinks he already knows."*
- *"If you want to improve, be content to be thought foolish and stupid."*

Not suggesting you become a Stoic philosopher, of course, but you may decide to embrace a few ideas as you take control of your sleep!

I wonder, as you become more Aesopian in the stories you share with friends and associates, whether you will see some common themes in the morals of Aesop's Fables and Lao Tzu's work, and the work of Epictetus, Seneca, and others. You are on a great journey if becoming a better storyteller, if even to your own mind, is what you desire. A true Renaissance fabulist! Again, for more insights on becoming more Aesopian in your thinking, consult my book, *The Magic of Aesop*, or simply reread the Aesop's Fables presented earlier in this book!

Let me share a good handful of mental programming and sleep-oriented Stoic affirmations that may help you reclaim a better sense of calmness and overall self-control. Stoic philosophy emphasizes self-control and fortitude. If it can help Vice Admiral James Stockdale survive seven and a half years at the Hanoi Hilton as a POW, it can help you sleep better! (Stockdale was the most senior naval officer held captive in Hanoi, North Vietnam. He was a firm admirer of Stoicism, and Epictetus in particular, whose lessons Stockdale attributed with supplying him strength to endure his time as a prisoner.)

Check off the affirmations that best resonate with you:

- ❑ My mind is unconquerable, and I free myself from distractions.
- ❑ I maintain my focus only on those things that I can control.
- ❑ I reign over myself. I reign over my reactions. I am in control of my emotions.
- ❑ My inner world is my palace, where I have absolute dominion

and control.

- ❑ I focus only on those things which uplift and enliven.
- ❑ I cultivate a sound mind in a sound body.
- ❑ I master each moment and I focus only on what is here and now.
- ❑ When any future event does come, I will always be ready for it.
- ❑ I am always in control of myself in any moment.
- ❑ I retain my sovereignty of lucid awareness.
- ❑ I take a moment before reacting, and find it easier to maintain control.
- ❑ I detach myself from exterior things, and unmoor myself from attachments. I free myself. I am free in myself.
- ❑ My mind is free, lofty, fearless, and steadfast.
- ❑ Nothing can subtract or add to my inner happiness.
- ❑ I find delight in my own resources, and I desire no joys greater than my inner joys.
- ❑ I am invincible. I am not affected by events.
- ❑ I retain control.
- ❑ I know that I have something in me more powerful and miraculous.
- ❑ I take a higher view of all things, and bear with them more easily.
- ❑ I hold myself responsible. I hold myself accountable.
- ❑ Everything in my life is my creation, and therefore mine to change, mine to improve, mine to exalt.
- ❑ I am steady and constant, I am looking inward.
- ❑ I seek only to improve myself. By improving myself I improve the world.
- ❑ I act always with decorum, in a disciplined and reasoned manner.
- ❑ I slow down and measure my every reaction.
- ❑ To be balanced, and august, is the greatest virtue.
- ❑ I remember that the contest is now.
- ❑ I now am at the Olympic Games.
- ❑ I will fulfill myself by attending to nothing except reason in

everything I encounter.

Wow! Lots of ground covered in the chapter and all prior chapters. Who knew that it would take so many words to share the deeper meaning of the four simple words *"I am sleeping now"*!

Important Insights from a Friend

We are at the point in this book (if you have not already looked ahead), where the next chapter focuses in quite specifically on how to help you get the sleep you deserve!

Before we get there, however, I would like to share a few insights from my friend and supporter, Dr. Michael Hathaway, who has been a true inspiration to me as a writer. Michael is the author of numerous books, including *The Everything Lucid Dreaming Book*, *The Everything Hypnosis Book*, and *It's Time to Simplify Your Soul's Code*. He is also the author of *Everything Happened Around the Switchboard*, the story of his family's Bryant Pond telephone company, the last old-fashioned hand-crank phone system in America, and the people who lived their lives around it. It is a fascinating story. The company's switchboard was donated to the Maine Museum, and his parents appeared on *The Tonight Show* with Johnny Carson decades ago!

Michael shared some insights with me in reviewing this book, specifically in support of your attaining sleep mastery. I want to provide them to you, as they add to the previous chapters.

Supporting the discussion in Chapter Four:

> I have found in my hypnosis practice that there are a lot of ex-military who have not been able to adjust to civilian life again because their sleep patterns in the service were connected to being hyper-aware of potential danger. In their current life, their sleep may be interrupted by a sudden sound or trying to fall asleep in an unfamiliar place. Setting intentions that if an interruption does occur they know that where they are now is safe. The practice of daily self-hypnosis can help retrain their minds for desired sleep results.

As you practice daily self-hypnosis in your new falling asleep strategies, remember the power of I AM as you set intentions.

Michael shares for Chapter Five:

> There is a technique of self-hypnosis for lucid dreaming known as dream incubation. As the subject prepares to fall asleep for the night, in a relaxed state they suggest to themselves that during the night they will become aware of a dream while they are sleeping. A good subject will actually be able to manipulate the dream to meet their goals set before going to sleep. This technique can also be used by suggesting that if they find themselves awake they can easily drift back into a pleasant restful dream.

Michael just shared an important secret to falling back to sleep!

He advises an insight for Chapter Six:

> When was first learning self-hypnosis, I was teaching full time during the day and playing piano in a lounge six nights a week. Needless to say, that created a problem for getting a good night's sleep, so I practiced suggesting to myself that when I went to sleep at night, I would wake in the morning feeling as if I had gotten a full eight hours' rest. I also would rest in the afternoon for a few minutes, suggesting to myself I would experience a good two-hour nap.

Remember, a nap and a hypnotic power nap are two different animals!

Michael suggests a great anchor for Chapter Seven:

> The daily practice of setting intentions for positive outcomes can be a valuable asset in forming positive sleeping habits. It starts with being conscious of the intentions you are setting. Your language to yourself is very important as it is sending out a message of what will come back to you. Negative language can attract negative results while positive language can attract positive results.

Remember, it is scientifically proven, and evidence-based: Our words determine the very destiny of our life, impact our immune system and ability to heal physically, mentally, and emotionally, and they impact the lives of others. Choose your words — for self-talk, and for external communication — very carefully. Words matter.

Finally, for this chapter (Chapter Eight):

> Back in the late 1980s I was struck by a car while crossing the street in a crosswalk. I found myself lying on the hot pavement with some bleeding coming from my mouth. I knew it was serious and I entered a state of self-hypnosis connecting to my belief that I was being watched over. Turned out I broke a leg, chipped a kneecap, and suffered a blow to the back of my head. Ten days in the hospital and then another ten days recovering from blood clots in my lungs, I was home with some pain medication. Fortunately, the doctor did not renew the medications and I would often wake with chronic pain. Again, I practiced self-hypnosis to help my sleep. Over time people with the gift of sight started asking what was standing behind me. I now truly believe that there is really something watching out for me, and many times a day I thank that source with heart-felt gratitude for watching over my journey as I set my intentions to do the best I can. What I am trying to say is that a positive belief system is, I believe, a major component of sleep.

Thank you, Michael, for sharing these insights. Dear reader, I hope you found them to add a new dimension to your learnings here. Now, onward, to the really good stuff, as they say! Sleep awaits, and we do not want to keep it waiting much longer.

CHAPTER NINE

Your Hypnotic Sleep Consultation Session

"Every day, in every way, I am getting better and better."
—Émile Coué

Think back to Chapter One for a moment. Do you recall that imaginary consultation with Hypnos, the Greek god of sleep? Pretend that you did, indeed, have that consultation and that your questions were answered. He shed some light on your personal situation and perhaps it triggered a few ideas.

Now, think back to those sleep-related questions posed to you in Chapter One. Maybe you want to go back to that chapter briefly to refresh your mind. Glance at them and focus on those that resonate most, and I wonder if you can begin to see your path forward?

This chapter is all about helping you to customize and fine-tune your individual sleeping habits and encourage you to experiment to find the optimal solution. Fair enough? I don't really want you to skip this information. It's too important. Decide what you are personally willing to change, as you read this chapter, and be aware of any resistance you may notice as you examine your pre-sleep routine. Where does the resistance originate? A fear? Worried about something? Stubborn about a particular suggestion and an unwillingness to change a current behavior?

You see, you are in the process of interrupting patterns of thought and habit, things that have crept into your life and created new subconscious routines. You are in the process of shifting your focus and presenting your mind with better thoughts and better questions so that your mind and body will follow your intentions and attention. As you begin to see and face your obstacles to sleep, whatever they may be for you, that welcoming path that leads you to better sleep begins to be revealed.

Before we go further, take a moment to relax right now... Please take a nice comforting breath right now. In through your nose, the best slow breath you can take. Hold briefly, and exhale through your mouth... and think *"Every day and in every way, I am getting better and better"*... at sleeping better... I fall asleep more easily and I am enjoying longer and deeper sleep through the night... better and better... Take in a nice comforting breath again right now... in through your nose, the best slow breath you can take. Hold briefly, and exhale through your mouth. As you inhale, think *"relax."* As you exhale, think *"calm"* ... pause and reflect on how it feels to take control of your emotions... and now... repeat this paragraph one more time!

It feels good to breathe and relax, while feeding your mind such a powerful autosuggestion. You are programming your mind for a self-fulfilling prophecy that your subconscious mind will help deliver for you, all based on the power of your intentions.

Let's try it again.

Every day and in every way, I am getting better and better. Take a nice comforting breath right now. In through your nose, the best slow breath you can take. Hold briefly, and exhale through your mouth. (And if you wanted to customize Émile Coué's famous phrase, tailoring it for use when applying it to help you sleep better — though no additional words are needed, necessarily — that's fine, too. You could say, for instance: *"Every day and in every way, I am getting better and better at preparing myself for sleep."*)

You are on your way! Practicing this phrase occasionally will lead to sleep success.

Training your mind and body to sleep requires a commitment that you are willing to make some changes in your pre-sleep routine. Don't have one? Yes, you do! It may be faulty, but your current habits, thoughts, and behaviors are your pre-sleep routine. It's now a matter of deciding what changes you are willing to make. After all, because conquering the sleeplessness is important to you, I am sure you are open to making changes. In my profession, we say that *nothing changes until something changes.*

Let's Not Get Too Aroused When It's Time for Sleep!

The goal here, with a smarter pre-sleep routine, and with better-directed focus and attention, is to calm the brain's reticular activating system. A calm reticular activating system will help you sleep better. The reticular activating system comprises an extensive portion of the brainstem. For the science-inclined reader, as Michele P. West and contributor Hillary Reinhold explain in West and Jaime C. Paz's book, *Acute Care Handbook for Physical Therapists*:

> The central brain systems are the reticular activating system and the limbic system. The reticular activating system (RAS) is composed of an ascending tract and a descending tract. The ascending RAS is responsible for human consciousness level and integrates the functions of the brain stem with cortical, cerebellar, thalamic, hypothalamic, and sensory receptor functions. The descending RAS promotes spinal cord antigravity reflexes or extensor tone needed to maintain standing.

> The limbic system is a complex interactive system, with primary connections between the cortex, hypothalamus, amygdala, and sensory receptors. The limbic system plays a major role in memory, emotion, and visceral and motor responses involved in defense and reproduction by mediating cortical autonomic function of internal and external stimuli.

More than you need to know for our purposes, but perhaps noteworthy. Think of your reticular activating system as an awesomely powerful mind tool within your body that you can direct, simply by the power of your intentions. Our intention creates our reality, and when your intention is to sleep, your RAS will assist you, when your intentions are congruent with your behavior. In other words, your mind and body are looking for alignment, matching your thoughts, feelings, imagery, and actions.

Here's a fun example for you. Chances are you can recall similar experiences. If I told you *not* to think about a pink elephant, what immediately comes to mind? Hmmm. Now try this: Look for a blue pickup truck today or tomorrow. Any make, any model. Let your subconscious mind take on that assignment so you do not have to think much about it. How many will you see, I wonder? Will they be Ford, Chevy, Dodge, Toyota, or another brand? Whatever the case, Your RAS will 'see' the blue pickup trucks effortlessly, without your conscious involvement.

Let me sneak this one into the conversation, and put your RAS to work for you: I want you to vividly imagine the color red. Red, red, red. Any shade of red, from pink to ruby red. It could be a stop sign, a taillight, a car, a traffic light, a tomato, a radish, or anything at all. Red, red, red. Now, let the red become for you, for the next seven days and maybe longer, an automatic subconscious reminder — all without even thinking about it — that you are becoming a master of your own life by mastering sleep. Imagine what that new you will begin doing when you once again enjoy sleep as you should be doing and will be doing! Imagine assigning your mind to focus on sleeping well.

The primary role of the reticular activating system is regulating arousal and awake–asleep transitions. Without launching into a course on neuroscience, it helps to be aware that your sleep routine impacts your reticular activating system and, more importantly, you can take action by the choices you make and the changes you decide to undertake when it comes to preparing for sleep.

The reticular activating system is used in virtually every part of our life. It is influenced by our predominant thoughts during our awake state and as we begin to move toward sleep, while our core beliefs are shaping our perception of the reality around us.

Here's a reality for you to embrace: You are on a journey toward developing your sleep skills!

Our conscious thoughts, and what we are focused upon, help the subconscious to deliver that reality, good or bad. As Lao Tzu said 2,500-some-odd years ago, pay attention to your thoughts! If you can conceive it, you can believe it, and you can achieve it. It is all based on what you are feeding your subconscious mind.

Back to your RAS.

The reticular activating system is involved in our fight or flight responses to the sense of fear, and it can become overactive by such things as post-traumatic stress, excessive worry, and your focus on negativity. The RAS controls your sleeping patterns and may become unregulated or overstimulated which, in turn, makes it difficult in getting to sleep and in remaining in the sleep state.

Of course, as we discussed earlier, it is best if you can learn to sleep without medications. If it should be the case that you do use medications now, however, know that as you learn to use relaxation techniques and self-hypnosis you may find that your need for medication fades completely. Let your RAS embrace that notion! Any changes in your sleep medication require the guidance of your physician. Your doctor can advise you. Please stay away from the scary and likely dangerous pharmacological recipes that are offered by insomniacs in social media groups.

To review – sleep and stress are firmly bound together, intertwined, with either one influencing the other. I think that's a given fact, right? Sleeplessness can lead to weight gain, for instance, and weight gain can lead to sleeplessness. Conversely, when you are less stressed, you sleep better and greet the next day with a new attitude. When you sleep better, you lower your stress as well.

With an open mind, with mental and actual rehearsal, that ever-elusive sleep will come back and you will be a changed person! CEOs have discovered (finally!) that a good night's sleep is important for all employees, including you! When you sleep well, among other benefits, you'll also lower your stress level.

Learning how to sleep well again requires discipline, patience, and belief on your part. You are training your mind and body to sleep. It's conditioning, as in any other skill-building exercise. So, because it is so important — sleep, that is — you need to make a decision that you will implement some new rituals and routines. Because you want to achieve this goal, decide you'll do the things that have been proven effective. Sleeplessness, as you know from reading and from life's experiences, comes from allowing your mind to busy itself with processing thoughts, ideas, worries, and fears — when what you'd much rather be doing, or what you're *trying* to do, is to calm your mind so that you can stop tossing and turning.

When it comes to sleeping, or with anything you are trying to accomplish, keep in mind that the mind follows the body, and the body will follow the mind. Think, act, and be a person who finds it easy to fall asleep. This means that you actually assess and adjust your pre-sleep routine to prepare yourself to fall asleep once you climb into bed. It also means, as a result, that you will easily fall back asleep should you arise to use the bathroom in the middle of the night. You might be surprised to discover that you will stay in your dream state while going to the bathroom (with the right self-talk), and slipping back into bed will anchor your sleep state. Getting back in bed can be an anchor to relax deeper. Pulling the covers up and hitting the pillow can be an anchor to fall back asleep again, and then closing your eyes along with a deep relaxing breath can be a third anchor that takes you back to slumber and dreamland.

Pre-Sleep: Conditioning Yourself for a Good Night's Sleep

"Now, blessings light on him that first invented this same sleep! It covers a man all over, thoughts and all, like a cloak; 'tis meat for the hungry, drink for the thirsty, heat for the cold, and cold for the hot. 'Tis the current coin that purchases all the pleasures of the world cheap, and the balance that sets the king and the shepherd, the fool and the wise man, even."
—Miguel de Cervantes, *Don Quixote*

We are certainly not tilting at windmills here. Natural, holistic sleep is at your doorstep! We are getting closer to the reality of you enjoying a better night's sleep.

I hope you are feeling better about your ability to take back more control, self-empowered to make the shifts in your thoughts, beliefs, and actions that will lead to new habits and ultimately change your brain! You see, every time you consciously practice new pre-sleep rituals and routines you are causing new neural networks to form in your brain. It's called neuroplasticity — the amazing ability to change the brain and our behaviors by changing our thoughts. Using our imagination to see, sense, and feel the mentally rehearsed pre-sleep activities you decide to adopt, we are telling our subconscious mind what we want it to deliver. So, begin to picture a good night's sleep, stop chasing it, and just let it happen. Trust the process.

I want to present a concept now that will allow you to take back control of your sleep, or any other aspect of your awakened daily life for that matter. And that idea is this — that your subconscious mind is much smarter than you may realize, always alert, and looking for congruence. When it realizes your desire for getting good sleep is real, and that you are willing to change your pre-sleep activities, it makes it happen. In the beginning, though, as with learning any skill, you must involve yourself consciously for the subconscious programming to occur.

Indulge me for a moment here as I ask you to tap into your wonderful imagination. I want you to step into the future briefly and begin to imagine how you will experience what it is like to sleep better. What will that be like for you? It's a multi-sensory experience. Feel it. Hear it. See yourself sleeping well. Enjoy it and hold onto it. Now, bring it right back to right now, in this moment. This is the new you emerging, having achieved progress toward your sleep mastery skills. Stay connected with the feeling and bring it right back to this moment now. Make it real in your mind and allow yourself to move in that direction with your habit change work.

Your Habitual Rituals and Routines for Best Sleep Hygiene Practices

Let's talk now about sleep hygiene for a bit. Researchers Jansson-Fröjmark, Evander, and Alfonsson, in their insomnia study titled "Are sleep hygiene practices related to the incidence, persistence and remission of insomnia? Findings from a prospective community study," found several sleep hygiene factors that affected both the insomnia sufferer as well as the non-insomnia diagnosed person dealing with sleep difficulty.

From the study:

> Sleep hygiene is a term that is commonly used to describe a set of behaviors or habits that may influence sleep quality. Sleep hygiene has often been viewed as having a contributing role for insomnia, which is for example apparent in diagnostic systems. The International Classification of Sleep Disorders (ICSD-II; American Academy of Sleep Medicine, 2005) describes inadequate sleep hygiene as a unique diagnostic entity highly relevant to sleeping problems. In the ICSD-II, inadequate sleep hygiene is defined as engaging in behaviors such as improper sleep scheduling, using sleep disturbing products, activating, or arousing activities close to bedtime, using the bed for activities other than sleep, and maintaining an uncomfortable sleep environment. The notion of inadequate sleep hygiene as a contributor to insomnia is also evident in that cognitive behavioral therapy (CBT-I), an evidence-based psychotherapeutic intervention for insomnia, typically incorporates sleep hygiene as a treatment modality.)

Among factors cited in their report, the following may have an impact on your own sleep preparation:

- Too much alcohol, especially close to bedtime.
- Nicotine.
- Caffeine late in the day or evening.
- The sleep environment; light and noise disturbances, primarily.

You can access the full text of the research paper in question at link.springer.com if you are so inclined. Sleeplessness and insomnia are widely studied and examined, as Google Scholar (a helpful and handy web search engine that indexes the full text or metadata of scholarly literature across a vast array of sources and topics) will prove. I shared the above to make the case for you taking a closer look at your sleep routine and with your greater awareness that you can mindfully make changes wherever you are so determined!

From a clinical hypnotist's perspective, we will review some of the same common-sense pre-sleep advice I share with my clients, to prompt you to start crafting your *own* pre-sleep strategy. You need to be aware of your current habits so a baseline for change can be established. From there, you will define and develop your own habitual success habits.

As I tell my clients who come to me for sleep improvements, brutal honesty is required if you are serious about sleeping better. Keep your mind open, because you've likely heard some of this advice before. This book, and the sleep techniques presented, are all centered on change work — tiny habit change, or transformational change, depending on the magnitude and scope of the issues. If you are simply too stubborn to change, are resisting change, lack confidence in your own abilities, or for whatever reason are unwilling to change what you do now in the time leading up to bed, then please reconsider. I say this from a place of compassion and kindness, and maybe a bit of much-needed tough love, too. Changing a few things may be precisely what is needed, so this is very important.

This change work is all about your personal authenticity and getting to know yourself better, all part of a quest to find greater happiness, abundance, and joy in your life, which God wants for you. The evidence-based success using hypnosis to resolve sleep issues requires that you remain open to change. Hypnosis is used to help the subconscious mind hear and apply appropriate and beneficial self-suggestions (or suggestions from the hypnotist in a clinical setting).

Ready for Some ZZZs?

Consider these sleep hygiene Zzz-Tips — presented in no particular order — and decide what's going to work best for you as you make your own personalized adjustments and change some self-sabotaging thoughts and habits.

There are countless lists of advice for helping you move toward enjoying a better night's sleep — and you have heard them all! There are countless books and other advice written by mattress companies, "sleep doctors," supplement companies, and pharmaceutical manufacturers that rehash "sleep hygiene" all leading you toward buying their various products. And there are countless online "insomnia support groups," as well, for people to commiserate and share their hopelessness. Maybe you have been disappointed by any or all of them. Here's hoping my list that follows will prove much more useful and beneficial!

I present these tips that follow as data points for you to consider as you ponder the habit changes, routines, and rituals you'll choose to adopt. Treat them as such. They are important, but keep your focus on the bigger picture.

Even though you were taught to never write in a book, this is *your* book! Please feel free to write in it. In fact, I encourage you to read through the list and then circle back and mark the most important and realistic suggestions for your unique situation. Then, circle back again and write down under those you've marked what kind of action you want to take.

#1: Let's go for cool, dark, and quiet. Shoot for 60–68°F, along with room-darkening drapes or shades. Think about how you can eliminate noise disturbances. And, if the noise disturbances are outside of your control, can you perhaps make them a positive anchor? Sleeping in a cooler room also helps contribute to weight loss, as well as enhanced mood when you awaken!

#2: Make sure your bedroom is as tidy as possible. Fresh linens. No books, food trays, and no pets on the bed. Your bed should be neat, and remember to make your bed when you arise.

#3: No food 2–3 hours before sleep. Make it a rule! Try it for the next 14 days and see if it makes a difference. Look into intermittent fasting, and look at your overall eating habits, especially portions!

#4: Limit sugar intake. No sugary drinks, or desserts late at night. Watch labels for any form of corn syrup. Sugar is everywhere. Maybe for a couple of weeks, you can cut your sugar consumption in half, then half again. Try it.

#5: Limit alcohol, especially before bed. This should be common sense, and if alcohol habits are a problem, decide what you are willing to change in this area of your life. I wonder if you can eliminate alcohol for a couple of weeks so you can notice how your sleep improves without it.

#6: Limit caffeine. No caffeine six hours before bed. Try green tea instead!

#7: No television at bedtime. Consider removing the TV from your bedroom. Your pre-sleep ritual may need attention if you are absorbed in television late at night. Plan on walking away from the boob tube — or any screen time — one hour before bed, for a week or two, to see how things change.

#8: No email, internet, or video games ONE HOUR before sleep. No blue screen. Best to eliminate blue light towards bedtime.

#9: Exercise 20 to 30 minutes a day but no later than a few hours before going to bed. There are conflicting studies about late exercise before sleep. You'll refine to suit your needs, but we want to shift the nervous system from arousal to calmness. Everyone is different. If you can fall asleep fast after a late-night workout, fine.

#10: Make a list of anything you don't want to forget overnight and keep a pad by your nightstand. I recommend doing this in your pre-sleep habitual rituals, but it's always a good idea to have pad and pencil within reach. If it's important, write it down so the idea is captured. Then drift back to sleep!

#11: No texting in bed or playing mindless games on your phone. Instead, read or do a crossword puzzle to relax. Unless you are awaiting important news from a loved one, silence your phone, and your so-called smartwatch, too, for that matter.

#12: No cellphone in bed. Place it well out of reach! Break the phone addiction habit. Again, silence all notifications.

#13: Set a schedule, going to bed and waking up at the same time each day. This is among the best conditioning you can do for returning to consistent, restful slumber. Sage advice. Consider it.

#14: Establish your relaxation routine before bed, as this book teaches, and as you add what works for you — try a warm bath, reading, or another relaxing routine. Remember the Relaxation Response taught earlier. Jumpstart it with calm, relaxed breathing a half hour before bed.

#15: Take a serious look at your media habits, especially television and various video streaming services, and decide to reclaim your life by limiting your time in that vast wasteland. I want you to have courage enough to make some changes in the context of your life, the time you have remaining on this planet.

#16: Make your bed. Doing so gets you up and about, moving, and makes you task-oriented, ready for what's next in your personal morning routine. As Navy SEAL Admiral William McRaven says in his famous speech, "If you want to change the world, start off by making your bed. You will come home to a bed that is made, that you made. And a made bed gives you encouragement that tomorrow will be better." Check out his YouTube video, seen by almost 14 million viewers. And, when your feet hit the floor, feed yourself a good strong positive affirmation, like: "How lucky am I to have the gift of today. Let me make today count!"

And there you have it, your sleep hygiene routine. Examine your current habits and beliefs about each of these points. Remember, your long-term success requires tiny habit changes and shifts in your beliefs and attitudes. Think baby steps, or incremental change. Slow and steady wins the race.

Let's tie this all together before we move to the next chapter.

- You have shifted from chasing sleep to inviting it to your doorstep. Even Hypnos, the god of sleep, has counseled you.
- You are adopting a new appreciation for sleep time, and your sleeping quarters are a sleep temple, just as Imhotep would have advised you.
- You have gotten to know thyself better, and have adopted new routines and new habitual rituals in your pre-sleep hour.
- You are aware of and are changing the stories you tell yourself so that sleep comes to you more easily each night. Your mind loves a good story. Let it hear your story about the transformational change happening within, as it unfolds.
- You can fall asleep as fast as any soldier in the U.S. Army using military sleep secrets that have been taught for decades, if not centuries!
- You take charge of your mind and body, using relaxation as a strategy for sleep, for health, and for improving the quality of your waking hours each day.
- You know how to clear the obstacles that hold you back from enjoying better sleep. You know how to fight the resistance

that pops up to defeat you.

- You have received advice from a 19th-century psychologist, Émile Coué, with an affirmation you can say daily: *"Every day, in every way, I am getting better and better."*
- You have learned the power of "I AM."

It's actually quite easy to fall and stay asleep, as you've already accepted as truth. You are doing your part to ensure success. Now it is time to put this to practice! Almost...

Oops! One more thing, and this is important. Very important.

As you might presume, hypnosis deepens your sleep experience. When you take control of the process and invite sleep to your pillow, in your pre-sleep routine, you are slowing your brain waves. Remember, I talked about the hypnagogic state, right below full consciousness. Slow-wave sleep (SWS), as it's called, plays a very important role in body health and restoration and promotes brain plasticity, our ability to change our brain with our thoughts, intentions, habits, movements, and our environment. While it is beyond the scope of this book to discuss in quite a lot of detail, know that we can rewire our brain and strengthen new neural networks, as touched upon previously. Neurons that fire together, wire together!

According to a study, "Deepening Sleep by Hypnotic Suggestion," from the University of Zurich, Switzerland:

> Slow-wave sleep (SWS) plays a critical role in body restoration and promotes brain plasticity; however, it markedly declines across the lifespan. Despite its importance, effective tools to increase SWS are rare. Sleep disturbances are highly common and present a major challenge for modern societies. Disturbed and insufficient sleep is strongly associated with several major diseases including hypertension, cardiovascular disease, obesity, depression, anxiety, bipolar disorders, and Alzheimer disease. In particular, slow-wave sleep (SWS) has proven vital for health and well-being, and slow-wave activity (SWA) during SWS benefits both the immune system as well as cognitive functions and

brain plasticity.

The study goes on to state:

> Furthermore, frequently prescribed sleep-inducing drugs typically hinder the occurrence of SWS, lose their efficacy during long-term treatment, have adverse side effects, and often are associated with a high risk of addiction. Thus, the development of efficient and risk-free approaches to improve sleep and particularly SWS are highly warranted. One nonpharmacological approach to improve sleep is hypnosis … [and there is] evidence for a beneficial effect of hypnosis on sleep disturbances and insomnias.

Further evidence that this holistic approach to sleep is the right one. No dangerous sleeping pills. No costly, silly gadgets or devices. No need for goofy apps on your phone, and no need for concoctions and unproven, unapproved supplements for sleep.

Change some habits. Learn to relax. Control the stress and anxiety in your life, turn in a good day, and hit the pillow with a clear mind.

CHAPTER TEN

The Magic of Hypnotic Sleep: Four "Secret Words" to Enter the Sleep Realm

"There is a time for many words, and there is also a time for sleep."
—Homer, *The Odyssey*

I agree with Homer! And there is a time for very few words, too! Four words, in fact: *"I am sleeping now"*!

These four words are the essence of the suggestions you will use to condition your mind for easy onset of sleep! The secret to falling asleep lies in your self-talk and in bringing yourself to the present moment, guided by your intention (to "go to sleep now").

Why did it take nine chapters to get to this point? Fair question if that's on your mind. What follows makes infinitely more sense if you have already read each previous chapter, as there is much foundational mind work in embracing these four simple words as the magical solution to your sleep woes.

Perhaps you are sleeping better already, with the learnings and discoveries found within these pages. Maybe you have started to investigate the merits of Tai Chi for sleep quality (which, by the way, I heartily recommend), or you have adopted the U.S. military's remedy for helping soldiers, sailors, and airmen to quickly fall asleep. Maybe you have filed those ideas to explore later, when your mind is aligned to do so. You will certainly sleep better tonight because of what you learn in this chapter alone.

I am sleeping now.

This is amazingly simple, and it works! I teach it whenever I speak, and with my private clients. I have taught thousands of people to fall and stay asleep using this technique.

It is because the subconscious mind is there to serve us, and you are consciously involving yourself in this shift of focus. The ego and the conscious mind become set aside in this process, allowing your mind to be directed by your words, and "I am sleeping now" simply becomes the truth in the moment.

The subconscious mind operates in the background, in the present moment, and it takes our language and intentions quite literally. It is *driven* by our intention, with a purpose to deliver whenever possible — so when your intention is to train your mind and body to sleep, your brain makes that happen. When your intention is to sleep, it is there to serve you. You simply need to (re)train your conscious mind and, just as I tell my golfing clients, step aside and let the subconscious mind do what it does when your intention is clear. In the case of the golfer, I instruct them to step aside, mentally, and let their mind and body swing the club. In our case here, the goal is to train your mind and body to sleep when it is time to sleep. You know how to sleep. It is simply a matter of allowing yourself to fall into the realm of slumber, undistracted by your conscious mind.

Could it really be that your positive self-talk can ease you into a good night's sleep?

Indeed it can. Your language choices program your mind to be in alignment and believe the words you have chosen to speak to yourself. Whatever you *believe*, is true to *you*. And your words play a huge role in programming your belief system, whether at sleep time (as is our current focus), or throughout any other time in your day or your life. Self-talk determines our destiny. It's time to stop the self-sabotage and self-defeating language that prevents sleep. Do not say, "I can't fall asleep," or, "I will try to fall asleep." And unless you have an official medical diagnosis of insomnia, stop calling yourself an insomniac and get out of those unhelpful forums on social media. Decide you are taking back the controls and unchain yourself from the negative imprints that have been, up until now, sabotaging your sleep!

I am sleeping now. Four magic words that bring sleep to you. Believe it, conceive it, and achieve it. Trust this process. It's easy to learn and apply, and you'll be wanting to take your new learnings and help others sleep better, too!

When you say these words silently and deliberately, perhaps adding a forced yawn or two, your body starts to respond. You shift to the present moment and start to call sleep to your bedside, inviting it to you as a fact. If you have made some changes in your daily living and in your pre-sleep routine, sleep will come and will stay throughout the night. You have decided what changes you will make so that sleep comes more easily.

HOORAY! Finally, we arrive at the heart of this book! Drumroll, please.

If I have not yet put you to sleep with my writing, let me do so with my time-tested and proven self-hypnosis technique that guarantees your sleep mastery. All I ask is that you practice this. You can access additional resources at www.iamsleepingnow.com to help you use this method for calming your mind and going to sleep.

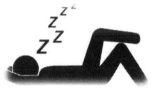

Let me walk you through the I AM SLEEPING NOW process with these instructions.

Here are the steps.

First, be done with the day's activity. You are in your sleep temple and ready for this healing rest. The intention is to climb into bed already relaxed. Your pre-sleep routine will make this possible. It is assumed you are following the recommendations laid out in the previous chapter and making a few changes to your habitual ritual.

Practice this mind–body conditioning each night, and mentally rehearse the positive outcome you seek — sleep! For support, watch the video at www.iamsleeping.com. You'll find it in the Resources section there. You'll also find support in the Facebook group with the same name.

Here's how you do it:

1. You are now in bed, comfortable and ready to go to sleep, or go back to sleep. (Lights out. No TV. No cellphones. No 'blue screen' activity for the past hour. No alcohol for three hours before sleep. No late-night meal. Do it.)

2. Take a nice deep relaxing breath... like the deep, relaxed breathing you were hopefully doing for a few minutes before getting into bed. Anticipate sleep. Continue to trust this mind conditioning journey as you put it into practice. Sleep will come. Continue to breathe and relax. As you inhale, think *"calm,"* and as you exhale, think *"relax."* I wonder if you can imagine your body responding. Soon your heart rate decreases, your blood flow increases, and your heart and lungs are pumping more oxygen to more places throughout your body. Every cell within you is smiling back at you.

   If you find your mind wanders, bring your focus right back to your breath. No worries. Breathe in... calm... breathe out... relax.

3. Get physically comfortable in bed. Settle in. Be as still as you can be, knowing (not hoping) that sleep is coming your way. Physical relaxation is first, then the focus is on mental relaxation. You will see that, with practice, this happens very quickly. You may want to do a quick progressive muscle relaxation 'body scan' to deeply relax physically, with practice and by using an anchor such as gently tapping the thumb and finger and thinking *"calm"* as you exhale. Yawn intentionally. With a little practice — and without trying too hard to perfect this, just let it come to you as it will — a few deep breaths and a quick anchoring as I've suggested will bring sleep to your pillow before you even say I AM SLEEPING NOW!

4. Now as you are comfortable and physically relaxed, take an-
   other nice, slow, deep breath… and softly say, "I am sleeping
   now."
   - Repeat ten times, using fingers to count as you say again,
     "I am sleeping now."
   - You will be asleep before you can count 5–7 times!
   - If you awaken in the night, repeat the phrase until you
     are back to sleep.
   - Do not allow your mind to wander. However, should this
     begin to happen, do not fight it. Rather, simply
     acknowledge the thoughts you are thinking and allow
     them to pass, as if you are ignoring them, and go right
     back to your mantra: "*I am sleeping now.*"

5. Train your brain, your mind, and body to anticipate sleep and
   condition yourself with this routine. It works, and it requires
   a little discipline and effort to master the skills. I have tremendous confidence in you. You've read this far, and you
   know that a holistic, chemical-free, drug-free approach is going to work for you, just as it does for thousands of others.
   Your mind cannot concentrate on more than one thing, and if
   you focus on "*I am sleeping now,*" you cannot focus on anything else. Try it!

Congratulations! You now have the technique. I AM SLEEPING
NOW will help you easily fall and stay asleep.

To review and simplify: After your new pre-sleep routine, hop
into bed already relaxed and breathing comfortably. Continue to
invoke the relaxation response. Get physically comfortable. Find
that favorite position in your comfy bed. Do a quick progressive
muscle relaxation 'body scan' to relax every cell in your body.
This should take but a minute or two with practice. (Anchor this
relaxed feeling by pressing your thumb and finger together, making a circle. Each night, use the anchor to instantly relax yourself.)

Now, get mentally relaxed. Set aside all negativity and doubt.
Do not *try* to go to sleep. *Go* to sleep, by reciting slowly, with a

calm relaxing breath in between, for a count of ten, "I am sleeping now." Trust the process. Know that you are conditioning yourself to fall and stay asleep.

Zzz-Tip: If you awaken for any reason, including a bathroom call, simply breathe deeply... in through your nose... exhale through your mouth... Deep relaxing breaths... and say, "I am sleeping now." This keeps your mind focused on your present-tense reality and prevents other thoughts. Stay in a light hypnotic trance and go back to sleep. This strategy keeps you from re-arousing your nervous system and brain functioning. Go back to sleep. Do not make any habitual trips to the kitchen. Do not do anything except hop right back into bed. Try to keep dreaming on your trip to the bathroom and back.

Success! Now, prepare yourself for the I Am Sleeping Now seven-day challenge in the next chapter, and plan to practice! But this first...

Additional Mind-Calming Strategies for Successful Sleep Mastery

Sometimes, when our racing mind is keeping us from mentally relaxing, additional strategies are required to distract the mind. The options are infinite and only restricted by your imagination. You'll begin to dream up all sorts of pleasant ways to distract your conscious mind so that sleep may cometh!

Pay attention when you are awakened in the wee hours.

Sometimes we are summoned by the spirit side of our being. Is God waking you in the middle of the night for a reason? Are spirit guides or your higher mind trying to get your attention? These were the ideas shared with me by Dr. Wayne Dyer many years ago, in a small group meeting hosted by one of my business consulting clients at the time. Dr. Dyer told us that it could be that God was awakening us for a reason, and that we need not always rush right back to sleep.

His words left an indelible impression on my mind, and inspired me to write the following poem a few years ago.

> In the quiet solitude of the dim pre-dawn light,
> Awakened by spirits on high and nearby.
> My heart sings "Here I am, LORD; it is I, LORD."
> Indeed, I have heard you calling in the night.
> The mysteries of life revealed by a dream, interrupted.
> Listen now, while fighting the calling of healing slumber.
> Be ever alert for the voice of God, ever present for those who
> hear it.
> The clarity of conviction brings alive the purpose of your
> being, by the grace He bestows.
> —Robert Martel

Be present with yourself and God. What do you have to fear? Here is another poem:

> The breezes at dawn have secrets to tell you
> Don't go back to sleep!
> You must ask for what you really want.
> Don't go back to sleep!
> People are going back and forth
> across the doorsill where the two worlds touch,
> The door is round and open
> Don't go back to sleep!
> —Rumi

As 13th-century Persian poet Rumi also tells us: "Put your thoughts to sleep, do not let them cast a shadow over the moon of your heart. Let go of thinking." His words echo another wisdom about waking up during the day, and planning on sleeping better at night, before life passes you by: "If your guidance is your ego, don't rely on luck for help. You sleep during the day and the nights are short. By the time you wake up your life may be over." Brilliant.

Prayer can be used as a sleep strategy.

Paying attention and *praying with intention* will help you sleep, if you are spiritual. So, instead of counting sheep, try this.

It has certainly worked for me, and many of my clinical hypnosis clients have reported an improved sense of calmness and inner peace, enabling sleep to arrive.

In Hebrew, it's called *kavanah*. It translates to "intention" or a "sincere feeling, and direction of the heart." It describes the essential nature of a worshiper's state of mind and heart. It is an absorption or emotional devotion to conversations with God. In prayer, it requires a devotional belief and sincerity, beyond mere recitation of prayer words. In my years of clinical hypnosis practice, while I am certainly not qualified to be a spiritual guide, I do encourage clients to take a full mind–body–spirit approach to making progress toward their intended goals, and, as appropriate, to invoke prayer as a strategy for inner calm and peace. It certainly helps with sleep.

As Lois Tverberg writes on biblical context, found online at the En-Gedi Resource Center:

> The prayers that Jesus and Paul prayed were a combination of spontaneous petitions and traditional prayers that were prayed at certain times of day. One of them that is still prayed today is called the *Amidah* or "Eighteen Benedictions." It is quite lengthy and consists of prayers for all the various concerns of the Jewish people. For thousands of years since Jesus lived, these petitions have stayed nearly the same.
>
> In contemporary Protestant culture, we tend to disdain rote prayer, preferring the intimacy of spontaneous prayer and feeling that a repeated prayer is empty and hollow. We wonder how a person could avoid just "going through the motions." The answer is a concept that the rabbis developed known as *Kavanah*. The word means "direction," "intention," or "devotion," and the idea behind praying with *kavanah* is that you set the direction of your thinking toward God, and toward praying the memorized prayer "with all your heart."
>
> A person who has *kavanah* focuses his entire being on prayer and is undistracted by the chaos around him. He

may have said the same prayer a thousand times, but his mind is sunk so deeply into the words that he is experiencing new insights and feelings from them today that he has never experienced before.

I share this to simply offer a perspective on a strategy that may prove to be powerful for you. I hope you find it useful, historical interest aside. You can, indeed, recite prayer with deep intention. Even a good sermon is hypnotic. Yes, prayer is hypnotic, if it's done well!

As David Reeves, President of the British National Register of Advanced Hypnotherapists (NRAH), shares in his popular article hosted by the Cuyamungue Institute's website:

> The ancient Hebrews used meditation with chanting, breathing exercises and fixation on the Hebrew letters of the alphabet that spelled their name for God, to induce an ecstasy state called *Kavanah*. (These ritualistic practices are very similar to auto-hypnosis.) In the Talmud, *Kavanah* implies relaxation, concentration, correct attention (motivation). People such as fire-walkers, and priests who used the religious practices of laying on of hands to make people faint onto the floor, are using auto-hypnosis to bring about an altered state of consciousness using suggestion and expectation.

(David is an archeological expert on sleep temples and the practices of the ancients — or as I call them, the sages of the ages.)

Prayer and autosuggestion are intertwined in the process of feeding our mind what it needs!

Aside from the benefits of a personal dialogue with God, let me present 'talking to God' or to your higher source as preparation for sleep. If you find yourself unable to fall or go back to sleep, then consider surrendering to the fact that perhaps — in the silence of the night — you may help invite sleep back with a short conversation with Him. Don't rule it out. If you are not a spiritual person, yet you recognize a higher being in your life, then simply be open to a conversation. These next few ingots of advice may help a faith-based person to find inner peace at bedtime.

Earlier in the book I spoke about the importance of the mind, body, spirit, and heart all working together. Prayerful intentions do make a difference. We move toward what is first real in our mind. Do you recall?

God's word can, indeed, bring you peace and comfort in the still of the night. It's certainly a better sleep solution than dangerous sleeping pills! Try on these Bible verses as a sleep aid. Different, I know, but comforting to those who believe.

> When you lie down, you will not be afraid; when you lie down, your sleep will be sweet.
> —Proverbs 3:24

> Peace I leave with you; my peace I give you. I do not give to you as the world gives. Do not let your hearts be troubled and do not be afraid.
> —John 14:27

> I lay down and slept, yet I woke up in safety, for the LORD was watching over me.
> —Psalm 3:5

> For He gives to His beloved sleep.
> —Psalm 127:2

> So don't worry about tomorrow, for tomorrow will bring its own worries. Today's trouble is enough for today.
> —Matthew 6:34

> In peace I will lie down and sleep, for you alone, O LORD, will keep me safe.
> —Psalm 4:8

Prayer, which is simply good communication and conversation with God, who is within you, can invite the peace and tranquility within your mind, body, and spirit that then enables sleep to come into your life when sleep is what's next. The Lord's Prayer, or your favorite prayer for your faith, are good choices. Personally, I will often recite the Hail Mary prayer. I find that to be useful in my pre-sleep calming time, or even as the last thing on my mind before drifting to sleep.

Prayer may not be for you, but if it is, regardless of your faith, there is another you may consider called the *Examen*, developed by St. Ignatius. For the prayerful, however, I do want to say a bit more. Scripture talks about it all, and yet the Bible's teachings on sleep is a topic that goes beyond our conversation here. I petition you to examine your sleep habits and your unique sleep requirements, and if you are slow to arise or sleeping too long, you may be depressed about life or using sleep to avoid facing life.

Sleeplessness is influenced by behavioral patterns, by beliefs and habits, and also, in part, by medical factors. It is all a matter of the nourishment of your soul — mind, body, and spirit working together. Do not ignore this big picture; it affects every aspect of your life, and you can improve your sleep by paying close attention.

The Examen (or Daily Examen) is a method of reviewing your day in the presence of God, which is helpful for finding peace within, and may help you if finding peace is an issue preventing restful sleep. Praying the Ignatian Examen is actually an attitude more than a method, a time set aside for thankful reflection on where God is in your everyday life. It consists of five basic steps, which are customizable to your unique experiences and your relationship with sleep, and which most people take more or less in order, and it usually takes anywhere from 5 to 20 minutes each day (or evening) to accomplish in total.

How to Pray the Examen – Per the Jesuits

1. Place yourself in God's presence. Give thanks for God's great love for you.
2. Pray for the grace to understand how God is acting in your life.

3. Review your day — recall specific moments and your feelings at the time.

4. Reflect on what you did, said, or thought in those instances. Were you drawing closer to God, or further away?

5. Look toward tomorrow — think of how you might collaborate more effectively with God's plan. Be specific and conclude with the "Our Father."

You may not find the above useful. But perhaps you do!

As part of your journey toward living a happier, more peaceful, and joyous life, I encourage you to explore the Examen prayer. (And every religion and culture has a similar version!) I took a slight risk in sharing it with you, but I find it helpful as a suggestion for clients who are so inclined, though I understand it may not be for everyone's palate.

Now, I do realize, of course, that not everyone reading this book takes a faith-based approach to their lives, and that some may be non-believers. For me, however, I approach my life and my clinical hypnosis work from a mind–body–spirit and heart-centered place. When we acknowledge that God is within us, and we also recognize the same is true for everyone else on the planet, we can begin to connect better with — as Dr. Wayne Dyer would say — our "Higher Source." You see, part of your sleep success lies in the inner peace you foster during your waking hours. Make sense? They are interrelated; sleep and awake.

Zzz-Tip: In Dyer's book, *Inspiration: Your Ultimate Calling*, he says: "There's a voice in the universe calling each of us to remember our purpose — our reason for being here now, in this world of impermanence. The voice whispers, shouts, and sings to us that this experience of being in form, in space and time, knowing life and death, has meaning. The voice is that of inspiration, which is within each and every one of us."

As I tell all my clients, I personally believe (whether they choose to or not) that God wants us to have abundance, joy, and prosperity in our lives, and that we have to do our part to bring more peace and joy into our life. Moving the ego and the conscious mind out of the way, so that the subconscious mind can do its job when sleep is what's next, is non-negotiable.

Dyer also says in this book that "we needn't presume to tell our Source what needs to be done to provide us with a happy, ful-filling life." He knows. With a settled and focused mind, listening to the silence in the space between our words, thoughts, and ac-tions, we allow the wisdom within us to shine. Yes, this helps with natural, peaceful sleep!

Imagine (Another) Imaginary Panel of Experts on Your Team

Earlier in this book, I presented the idea of a consultation with Hypnos, the god of sleep (and also the inspiration in naming the phenomenon called hypnosis). Do you recall?

Were you able to imagine yourself traveling back in time to meet with Hypnos? What did you learn about yourself? Go back to that section of the book if need be.

Using that same wonderful and creative imagination within, let's add to the panel of historical sleep experts. Let's bring some of the well-revered Stoic philosophers and other notables to the table.

Imagine we've got Epictetus, Seneca, and Marcus Aurelius, plus Pythagoras and Aristotle at the table as well, along with our old friends Aesop and Hypnos, too, for good measure. Let's invite all of them to help you sleep better.

Put yourself in a very light hypnotic state by taking a few re-laxing deep breaths and count down, from 7 to 1, releasing any stress and tension as you go... as if you are descending down to that room where you find this illustrious panel of sleep experts from the past — the sages of the ages — there to help you see new insights, feel new feelings, and relax into the knowing that sleep comes easily for you. Simply say your favorite "I AM" affirmation as you think about the onset of sleep.

So, now, as we wrap up this leg of the journey toward better sleep, I hope you can begin to adopt a new relationship with sleep.

Let's put it all together:

- Imagine your bedroom as a revered place — your sleep temple.
- Break the mold of old sleep habits and create new habitual rituals that work for you.
- Invest in yourself emotionally, mentally, physically, and spiritually.
- Manage your stress and anxiety, and learn to live in the present moment.
- Rule out a medical diagnosis of insomnia and speak to your doctor about ending your health-harming pharmaceutical sleep medication prescriptions.
- Focus on sleeping better, not on sleeping poorly. This means leaving the insomniac groups on social media, as misery loves company. Own your new journey of healthy, holistic sleep. Focus on what you want, because where the attention goes, the energy flows.
- Do not chase sleep. Let it come to you naturally. Funny thing, this thing called sleep. The more you chase it, the more it evades you.
- Relax by mastering Benson's "Relaxation Response," which is just simple breathing.

CHAPTER ELEVEN

Your Seven-Day Sleep Improvement Challenge

"Never give in, never give in, never, never, never, never in nothing, great or small, large or petty, never give in except to convictions of honor and good sense."

—Sir Winston Churchill

Winners never quit. You are a winner. You will win by successfully mastering sleep!

The fact that you are reading this page speaks volumes about your determination to win the game and sleep well again. You've come this far, and I am certain you are already sleeping better or anticipating a restful sleep tonight.

Wisdom of the ages says it takes 21 days to change a habit. Not true with hypnosis!

In seven days, if you follow this sleep challenge, you will be sleeping much better. Yes, you may notice your sleep technology reporting better sleep, but I prefer to forego the fancy gimmicks and rely on the amount of energy and the *joie de vivre* you feel when you arise the next morning. What I mean to say here is that all of the new technology in the world is great. But what really matters is how you feel each morning, as you sleep better and better each night, as you master the skills of sleeping well.

I want you to apply that same mental toughness you bring to your daily life when it's important and you set the intention to see it through to completion.

Sleep is at your doorstep!

In fact, you are on your way to enjoying a seven-night journey to the best sleep of your life — assuming, of course, that you embrace the learnings presented thus far and you practice, practice, practice! Sleep will come easier each day. I promise.

As the Mayo Clinic says, regarding sleep:

> *Ease into sleep.* Setting aside a little time before bed for relaxation can help you transition into sleep. Try deep breathing, progressive muscle relaxation, gentle stretching or guided imagery to help focus your attention away from worries and into the present. If your busy mind keeps you awake, jot down your thoughts in a journal or on a pad of paper by your bed.

At this point, I am confident that you have all the necessary sleep mastery knowledge to put into practice. Sleep is a revered and precious phase of your life, and you embrace it now, likely more so than in the past. Your pre-sleep routine has been examined. Your habits — both good, and those not so good — have been reviewed and you have decided which ones require your attention.

***Success* is at your doorstep as well!**

There is another quote I would like to share, often attributed to Churchill: "Success is the ability to move from one failure to another without loss of enthusiasm." As I teach my clients, there is no such thing as failure except failure to try, to act, to move toward your goal. Every time your head hits the pillow, you create a new opportunity for a successful night's sleep.

Good habits help you break the old habits that were in the way of sleep, and all self-sabotaging beliefs, thoughts, and behaviors are being examined as you now welcome sleep back into your life in a big way!

Now, let's put your plan in place.

It starts with knowing like Yoda would know and to do this in the present tense. *Know*, not hope. *Do*, not try. There is only do, or do not.

Each day for the next week, when you arise from whatever

sleep you experience, I want you to say the following (pick one):

- *I am okay. I am conditioning myself to once again sleep well!*
- *Every day and in every way, I am getting better and better (at falling and staying asleep).*
- *I sleep well and awaken refreshed.*
- *I am keeping an open mind as I condition my mind and body to be calm, relaxed, and tranquil as I reconnect with my sleeping state.*
- *I AM SLEEPING NOW* (preferred version, but your unique phrase will also work!)

Keep in mind that the key to your success in adopting any new skill is to concentrate, with greater awareness, bringing your full attention to the task at hand. Each time you hop into bed, focus with a new mindset, and be honest with yourself in making the changes you know you ought to make, secure in the knowledge that you are taking back control of your sleep time routines. Commit to a week as you sincerely train your mind and body to allow you to enjoy what may be eluding you now.

Zzz-Tip: Each day for the next week or two:

- Go to bed at or near the same time each night and awaken by alarm clock at the same time each morning, if possible. Cell-phone out of reach.
- As you wind down, examine your day. Did you awaken with more positivity? Regardless of circumstances, a positive outlook is a choice. Greet the day as the gift that it is, and decide to be happy, grateful, and productive. Make a difference in the lives of others, with compassion and kindness.
- Thank yourself for the positive changes you've made with regard to your pre-sleep routine. (You know what changes to make — if you are willing to do so.)
- Relax prior to getting into bed by taking 30 minutes to unwind without television, social media, email, or any 'blue light' from technology. Begin to welcome sleep time into your life as "what happens next" in your day. The goal is to climb into bed

already in a relaxed state; blood pressure is down, heart rate is lowered, breathing is relaxed. Set yourself up for success. (And do not allow yourself to say, "I can't" — which really means you *won't*.)

- Remember to eat properly and shift to a healthier relationship with food. Decide to agree not to eat for at least two hours before bed. You can do it. Changing eating habits and letting go of alcohol for these seven days is a good idea. Think about giving alcohol a rest if it's a part of your life at the moment.

Day One

Okay. You are embracing this idea that self-hypnosis is going to do the trick for you and help you ease into a good night's sleep. Great! Stay open to the process. Use positive self-talk, and decide to *invite sleep to come to you.* Relax into the knowing that this works for others, and will work for you as well. Do not *try* to go to sleep. *Go* to sleep. (If you are taking prescribed medications, talk to your doctor about your desire to wean yourself off of them. You and your doctor can best decide how to ultimately say goodbye to sleep meds!)

Before you hop into bed, take five to ten minutes to simply breathe slowly, deliberately, deeply, to jumpstart the relaxation response. Your mind and body will become calm as you set the intention to do so. Heart/brain congruence is happening.

Once in bed, having already started to relax during your pre-sleep routine, here is a review of the process:

- Get comfortable in the position you like best for sleeping.
- Focus on physical relaxation first. Use a brief body scan technique or use the index finger and thumb anchor to help you be still, relaxing every muscle in your body. Simply allow them to all relax, together, at once.
- Now, mentally relax using the techniques presented in Chapter Ten. As you learn to take control and bring your focus and attention to falling asleep, you'll begin to develop your own 'mental field trips' to calm your mind.

I suggest, at this point, you use what's called the light switch self-hypnosis technique as you say to yourself, *"I am sleeping now."* The light switch technique is based on eyes opening and closing, taking a nice relaxing breath in between. Alternatively, you can use the finger-counting method, saying *"I am sleeping now"* as you keep your eyes closed, breathing slowly and deeply, repeating for the count of ten (if you get that far!).

Remember, this is a mind and body conditioning process. Expect to enjoy a better night's sleep. You may respond quickly, but anticipate a few days of conditioning. Should you awaken during the night to use the bathroom, focus on relaxed breathing as you gently repeat to yourself, *"I am sleeping now."* Then, return to bed immediately. You may even experience the same dream state you were enjoying!

Action item: Examine your pre-sleep habits. What have you changed? What are you stubbornly refusing to let go of, despite knowing it may be impacting you negatively? What new habit or change have you decided to add to your pre-sleep routine?

Day Two

Okay. You are on your way to mastering your sleep skills! Review the Day One recommendations above. Challenge yourself to stick with it, following the same process, with an openness that supports your intention, and practice this new-to-you I AM SLEEPING NOW method.

This is the second night of using this new approach. Yes, it is amazingly simple. It requires your discipline and your awareness as you continue to practice your sleep mastery skills.

Action item: During the day, take a moment to pause and enjoy a few nice deep relaxing breaths. Then say to yourself: *"Every day and in every way, I am getting better and better at falling and staying asleep."*

When you do get to bed, say "I am sleeping now," for only ten times — if you get that far. Be aware of self-talk, as you program your mind for positivity and expectancy. You are moving toward sleep mastery and it requires belief in your own abilities to feed yourself good suggestions as you end your day.

Day Three

Hopefully, you are already sleeping a little better, maybe a whole lot. Follow the Day One recommendations. If you notice your mind racing, and it seems like thoughts are occupying your mind, take back control by giving your mind something else to do while you progress into hypnagogia, the alpha brainwave state.

If you find yourself still awake after 5–10 minutes, try this: Allow your eyelids to feel heavy, as you count from 10 down to 1, imagining a staircase. Anticipate sleep as you arrive at the bottom step, gently tapping your index finger and thumb, very gently, and saying softly, "I am sleeping now." Make sure your room is cool and comfortable, and any stresses of the day are set aside using ideas we've discussed.

Day Four

Reread and follow again the above guidance. Examine your pre-sleep routine. If you are still awake, no worries. Anticipate sleep coming right to your bedside soon! Stop trying to go to sleep. Imagine a marker board with a circle drawn, and the letter 'A' in the center of it yet not touching the circle. Now, imagine gently erasing the letter 'A' and slowly drawing the letter 'B', and slowly, with a nice relaxing breath in between and thinking *"calm,"* continue to draw the rest of the alphabet if you can! Maybe by the letter 'F' or the letter 'G' or so, you'll be slipping into slumber. I doubt you'll get to the letter 'Z' but you will start to Zzzz! Stay with this mind-clearing exercise. It works!

Zzz-Tip: Here is another technique you might try, offered by a client. Sophia had come to me for hypnosis to help her sleep better. In the process of working with her, a pleasant, happy-place sort of memory arose in her mind. She recalled visiting her aunt's farm back in Belarus and picking raspberries as a child. It was a very happy memory for her. Imagine (assuming you like raspberries) slowly, patiently, picking only the ripest, juiciest of berries, one at a time, please. Gently pick one and place it in your basket. Hey! Don't eat them! Imagine there are 100 berries in all, right in front of you in the berry bushes, easily within reach. As you pick them, count backwards from 100 as you go along, counting each berry you pluck, and taking a slow deep breath as you go. As you pick them, however, the berries seem to get harder to see so you simply stop picking at some point, tired perhaps, and so you lie down in the raspberry patch and go to sleep.

I've used this technique with clients ever since Sophia shared her memory. She and I turned it into a nice mental exercise that worked not just for her but for others as well. Maybe it will help you also! She'd be happy to know that it did. Try it, or a variation.

Day Five

Chances are that you are already sleeping quite naturally. Continue to maintain a positive mind about sleep. Be aware of habit changes you are wanting to make and are making progress on, and those habit changes that you simply are not willing to make right now.

I want to invite you to go to the beach, in your mind, if you like the beach! Otherwise, pick your favorite outdoor scene, a place where you might imagine yourself being, enjoying all there is to experience. Imagine this place as you experience all of the sounds, smells, observations, and feelings of deep relaxation. Stay in that place as you invite sleep to your bedside. Enjoy that scene as you drift down deeper, slowly entering the sleep realm. Maybe you can imagine a small grain of sand between your thumb and finger, with you being focused on the feeling of the sand, feeling its unique edges as you slowly roll it between your fingertips. Careful not to drop it! Yawn a couple of times and say, "I am sleeping now."

Day Six

Recognize that this is a process, and it works! "I am sleeping now" is a positive, present-tense autosuggestion that your mind, body, and spirit will embrace — so long as you discard disbelief and negative self-talk. Eliminate the phrase "I can't sleep" and be willing to face what might be the real cause of your sleeplessness. Change it.

Day Seven

Congratulations! By this point, or maybe even sooner in the process, you have enjoyed a better night's sleep and hopefully you feel great! You'll find a video on the 7-day sleep challenge explained, at www.iamsleepingnow.com. It is in the resources you'll receive.

If you find that you are struggling with the above 7-day challenge, and the online resources are not helping, something else might be going on. Get in touch through the website and request a consultation. As I said at the outset, I am on a mission to help you sleep better.

Zzz-Tip: This seven-day challenge is not so much a challenge but a program for you to follow, especially if you are not making the full progress to sleep mastery. We all have sleepless nights now and then. Return to this as needed, reread Chapter Nine and Chapter Ten, and revisit the questions found in Chapter One as well. The U.S. military's method may work for you, which is similar to the I Am Sleeping Now method anyway. Practice the relaxation response and the "I AM" affirmations. Maybe the biblical angle helps. Keep an open mind and, of course, see your doctor. Stay out of those online insomnia "support" groups, as they are just filled with people who prefer to wallow in their own misery. Sorry. It's true. Get out of those groups!

CHAPTER TWELVE
Final Thoughts and Next Steps

"You will never do anything in this world without courage. It is the greatest quality of the mind next to honor."
—Aristotle

The magic is happening. You are on your personal journey to sleep mastery!

Thank you for reading this book and for allowing me to be a part of your journey. The journey continues as you forge ahead, mastering sleep and letting it once again become a natural experience. You've showed courage in wanting to master sleep naturally, using your mind, and I honor you for facing all that you needed to examine as you took back control. Keep it up!

What's next for you? As Aristotle suggests in his quote, above, I wonder how you'll continue to honor yourself? Here's a hint to consider: Focus on that idea mentioned in this book — that you should live your daily life well, to the best of your abilities, and that with confidence you can do anything you put your mind to and turn in a good day. Be optimistic about the following day, count your blessings and gifts, and share your talents and passions with the world. Sleep better to live better!

As you put your new sleep strategies in place, I wonder how your life will improve? What will change for you? What will it be like to experience a more refreshed, well-rested self each day?

I am certain that your friends, co-workers, family members, and loved ones will respond positively to your new refreshed self! Your relationships, your charisma, your influence as a relaxed being will all improve, not to mention your sex life will improve, too!

We all need sleep, and hopefully I have taught some easy, drug-free, holistic, mind-powered techniques for your improved health and well-being.

You know that quality sleep is imperative and is vital in the performance and quality of our daily lives, as mentioned throughout this book. So, it is a safe bet to assume you'll be doing more, feeling happier and healthier, and perhaps having a sense of relief that you have taken back control of an issue that used to plague you. You now have the tools to fall and stay asleep easily and quickly.

It's essential that you embrace a change in thoughts and habits in order to end the sleep struggle. Be mindfully aware of your own resistance to the habits that need to change. Decide that a relaxed and matter-of-fact resilience, determination, and certainty will help you make the tiny habitual changes that will lead to your successful outcome. Focus on the process of relearning how to fall and stay asleep. Trust the process of your mind and conditioning. Sleep will come! It will arrive naturally, as you allow it.

There will come a time real soon, if it has not occurred already, when you begin to forget that sleeping was ever an issue at all. Magically, effortlessly, and quite automatically in the present moment, day-to-day, you sleep well each night. It is a self-fulfilling prophecy.

Remember to commit to use the proven and effective Émile Coué self-programming autosuggestion: "Every day, in every way, I am getting better and better."

Let your subconscious mind fill in the rest of that sentence according to your intentions.

Keep the following tips in mind, too, as a reminder. As stated earlier, you will find that right balance of daily activity, mindfulness, attitude, and pre-sleep rituals that work best for you:

- Sunlight during the day helps you sleep better each night. Get out and enjoy the fresh air, even on a cloudy day. The sun shines through the clouds!

- Relaxation using self-hypnosis will facilitate easier sleep. Commit to a daily self-hypnosis habit for 5–10 minutes.
- Exercise during the day but not too close to bedtime. Go for a walk or plan regular exercise, two common solutions for helping you sleep more soundly.
- Alcohol should be minimized or avoided. If you will not stop alcohol use, consider refraining from it for a few hours prior to bedtime.
- Caffeine should be limited late in the day. Get in the habit of drinking less caffeine as the day progresses, perhaps setting a rule of none after 3 p.m. or so.
- Stress-reducing techniques will contribute to sleep quality.

As you move forward, please keep this promise to yourself: that you will continue your journey within to better understand your relationship with sleep, embracing it with reverence, and finding that optimal amount of sleep time that helps you bring your best game to life each day and to live a happier, more joyful and abundant life.

Revisit the 23 questions posed in Chapter One. If there is anything still blocking you from enjoying better sleep, and your sleep doctor has not produced an insomnia diagnosis, then these questions, and a review of Chapter Nine, should help.

Keep this pearl of wisdom in mind also, for in your warm and authentic heartfelt self, I know you know this: At the end of each day, as you live your life fully and sincerely, think to yourself, *"What has this day brought me, and more importantly, what have I given to it?"*

There is an Irish proverb that comes to mind as well: "A good laugh and a long sleep are the two best cures for anything."

I wish you plenty of both in your life!

I hope this book has helped you move toward sleep skill mastery. Thanks, again.

Goodnight! Sweet dreams.

Keep in touch.

Please go to www.iamsleepingnow.com to download an audio that I have created to help you sleep better, and to access additional resources that help you use the power of your own wonderful mind using self-hypnosis.

BONUS CHAPTER

Sleep Your Way to Success with an Energized Life Force!

"There is a vitality, a life force, an energy, a quickening that is translated through you into action, and because there is only one of you in all of time, this expression is unique. And if you block it, it will never exist through any other medium and it will be lost. The world will not have it."

—Martha Graham

Connect with your life force. Isn't that partially the purpose of getting a good night's sleep?

I titled this chapter as I did because, let's face it, as I mentioned earlier in this book, there should only be two purposes for going to bed. One of them is sleep, and the other is intimacy — or more directly, sex! And, true to the title above, a consistent good night's sleep does help one's overall success in life. (Note: And when I say "sleep your way to success," I'm of course referring to sleep in the literal sense!)

Sex and sleep are part of your life force!

Now that you have learned to love your bed again and have advanced your journey toward sleep mastery, this chapter might help you learn to love in bed again, well-rested. Love your bed, and love *in* bed, I say! Let's focus on your libido.

I invited Kaz Riley, an award-winning hypnotherapist and internationally recognized expert on intimacy, to contribute this bonus chapter. You see, once you are sleeping well again, you can enjoy intimacy at a much deeper level. And the oppositive is equally true as well, that better sex leads to better sleep. (These

topics of discussion lie slightly outside my area of expertise, however — which is why I invited Kaz to weigh in.) Sex and sleep are
two deeply connected experiences. We need both!!

Please enjoy Kaz's contribution to both your sleep journey and
your love life. You'll find her contact information, along with a
special audio download as well, in the Resources section over at
www.iamsleepingnow.com.

Better Sleep Leads to Better Sex

By Kaz Riley

You often do something else in bed other than sleep — sex. It's a
little ironic; one is peaceful and quiet, your heart rate slow and
steady, your blood pressure drops as you slumber, and you restore your energy levels ready for another day. The other makes
your heart pound, your blood pressure soar, can be very noisy,
and can leave you feeling really quite exhausted. But there are
many things sleep and sex have in common other than putting a
spring in your step and sending you out of the door whistling
with a glint in your eye the next day. Sleep and sex both send feel-
good hormones and neurotransmitters whizzing around your
body and both are essential to your libido, or life force as I like to
call it. Your life force is a collection of things that give you drive
in life. The things that motivate you, interest you, enrich your life
experience, your sensuality, playfulness, eroticism, sexual drive
and pleasure. They are the things that make you feel happy and
satisfied with life and drive you forward to embrace different experiences, seek out opportunities and take pleasure in all of that.

Now for those of you that don't know, the author of the book
you are reading, the wonderful Bob Martel, has a passion for pi-
loting hot air balloons, which is the perfect analogy and one I use
often to explain your life force and libido.

Imagine for a moment that your life force in its entirety is like
an enormous, beautiful and vibrant hot air balloon. It needs fuel-
ing with hot air to expand, fill up, and take off to great heights, so
that you can soar upwards in life.

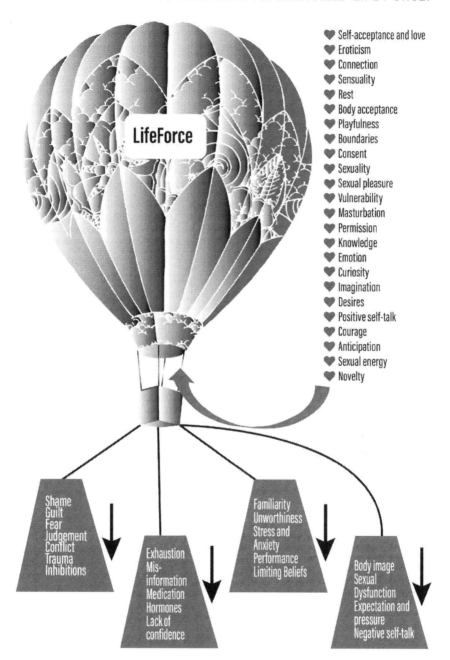

Image © copyright, Kaz Riley. All rights reserved.

Now imagine that hot air needed is made up of a collection of ingredients essential for your vitality, the "feel good's" and the "in good health's" that drive you forward in life. Confidence, sensuality, laughter, ambitions, successes, connection, a healthy body, good body image, sleep, and SEX! all being fired into the hot air balloon, causing it to fill, expand and take off. Now imagine you look over the side of the basket and you see there are sandbags weighing down the balloon, preventing it taking off. The sandbags are your doubts, anxiety, shame, stress, grief, health issues, feeling bad about yourself, negative self-talk, exhaustion, and many more of the things in life that can weigh you down. You have to let go of and disconnect the sandbags, so you can rise upwards feeling great, full to the brim with your vibrant life force. So how does this relate to sleep? If you don't get enough good quality rest and sleep not only does that stop the balloon becoming filled enough for a safe and exciting flight, but it also adds extra weight to the sandbags. It stops you rising (no pun intended) due to your life force being dampened and holds you back. Lack of sleep, or not getting quality sleep, makes stress worse, doubts bigger, health issues more intense. It weighs you down in life. Think how heavy you feel when you are exhausted, overwhelmed, and your body aches with fatigue; it can feel like you are wading slowly through treacle and stuck. Sleep is also essential for the "hot air" of your balloon to have enough heat for it to lift. Lack of sleep essentially "cools" the air, you feel less confident, your senses close down, you're, too tired to laugh and your sense of humour takes leave. Sleep, or the lack of it, has a huge impact on every aspect of your life, and that includes your sex life. Your life force is not the only part of your sex life that can be positively or negatively affected by sleep. Getting enough rest also balances the hormones needed for connection, desire, arousal, and even sexual function.

Anxiety and depression, both side effects of insomnia and sleep deprivation, are known to cause sexual dysfunction for a variety of reasons. When the body becomes stressed through exhaustion, the brain begins to suppress the production of sex hormones such as estrogen and testosterone. This, in turn, increases the production of stress hormones such as cortisol. This shift in hormone levels can lead to decreased life force, fertility issues, erectile dysfunction, anorgasmia, and a mismatch in mental arousal and physical response (the mind is all in but the body shouts "I need sleep!"). It can also cause you to not enjoy sex as much, which eventually makes it less important to you and takes away from your life force.

It's not all about biology, though. Lack of sleep and exhaustion simply make people too tired to have, or more importantly to enjoy, sex. So sex becomes a chore, something else to do on a list of tasks, which stops people being playful, erotic, and indulging fully in the experience. This makes sex become predictable and dull and lacking in novelty. This means we don't produce the same amounts of dopamine that drive our "wanting" system. Tiredness is the number-one cause reported by individuals or couples who have lost interest in sex. The good news is that a 2015 study conducted at the University of Michigan Medical School found that the longer people slept, the more they were interested in sex the following day. So, if you get more sleep, it's likely it will have a very positive impact on your sex life, and your sexual pleasure will improve. This is often a revelation to my sexual freedom hypnosis clients, when I tell them that if they are exhausted, first focus on getting better sleep, and then to focus on sex.

More Good News: Sex Helps You Sleep

A healthy sex life can help you sleep better, which in turn improves your sex life further and your life force. The connection between them is an important one.

Sex before sleep can help improve the quality of your sleep. When we have good sex — so, not when you are too exhausted to engage and connect — your body releases endorphins, which eases anxiety and helps you relax. Sex also releases oxytocin, a hormone known as the "love hormone," which has numerous benefits to your body and mind, including feeling connected and

191

bonded with another person. So getting great sleep can improve your relationship. We also release these hormones when we orgasm, either through sex or masturbation — so you don't need a partner, and can get these wonderful benefits even if you sleep alone — and science backs this up.

"This hormone [oxytocin] among many other feel-good hormones has been said to act as a sedative to reduce the time it takes to fall asleep," says Michele Lastella, Ph.D., a sleep scientist at Central Queensland University in Adelaide, Australia. Lastella conducted a survey of 460 adults between the ages of 18 and 70. Participants were asked about their sex lives and sleep habits. 64 percent of respondents said they slept much better after having an orgasm shortly before bed, likely due to the release of oxytocin and other endorphins that accompany orgasms.

How to Improve Your Sleep and Sex Life

To ensure your body is ready for sex,

- Aim for seven and eight hours of sleep each night.
- Notice what fills your life force hot air balloon, do the fun things in life that make you happy, it will have a positive impact on your desire, eroticism, sleep and outlook on life.
- Release the sandbags that are holding you back- negative emotions such as stress, shame and guilt can keep you awake at night and impact on your sleep and your sex life.
- Leave your phone out of the bedroom. If you and/or your partner spend each night staring at your phones in bed, you likely won't be in the mood for sex.

Sex or simply orgasms before sleep will help you sleep better, which in turn can improve your sex life even further, it's the perfect win–win. While a happy sex life isn't the only way to get a good night's sleep, getting sufficient sleep certainly is vital for your body and mind to be ready for sex. Getting enough sleep ensures you have both the energy and stamina to have sex, and enjoy it, whilst sleep also allows your body to regulate its hormones to be ready to experience that loving feeling.

Kaz Riley is an award-winning and leading international hypno-tist, hypnotherapist, and hypnosis educator. She is recognized as an expert in the fields of sexual freedom, sexual dysfunction, and kink-friendly hypnotherapy. She has an excellent international reputation for both her work with clients and her specialist train-ing and mentoring programs for hypnotherapists. Kaz is the founder and creator of Sexual Freedom hypnosis, which is now taught across the world. You can find out more at sexualfree-domhypnosis.com and kazriley.com. Kaz's book, *Woman: How to Find, Understand and Embrace Your Sexual Pleasure*, is available now.

ADDITIONAL RESOURCES

Tools to Help You Sleep Better by Living Better

5-Minute Relaxation and Self-Hypnosis Exercise
Change your thoughts and you change your life!

I created this exercise for my clients, to help them stay calm, relaxed, and in control in any situation. It is my strong belief that, if one can control their emotional state while awake and moving through their daily life, then it only helps one to sleep better.

Get ready to treat yourself with a wonderful gift, designed to help you stay in charge of your emotions in any situation by training your mind and body to remain calm, relaxed, and in control. This little routine, as basic as it seems, has helped thousands of people to maintain their sanity and emotional control in an otherwise stressful situation. Once you learn how to take control and stay in charge of your emotions, you will have considerably more influence over the outcome of the situation, or you may simply calm your own anxiety by learning how to relax. With practice, as you train your mind, with a commitment to program yourself for success and with less stress in your life, this exercise will quickly bring you to a state of calm relaxation and serenity. It may become habit-forming!

Find 5 minutes each day to practice this exercise. Over time, you'll be amazed at the positive impact it has on your ability to stay calm and relaxed in any situation. You'll command the moment. Do it early morning, at lunchtime, or at the end of the day. It can be either at work or at home (at home if possible), any time you've got a bit of quiet time to yourself. Closing your eyes eliminates any visual distraction, making this tool even more powerful. Here we go...

1. Close your eyes (once you know this "script"). Allow yourself to take a nice long deep breath, exhale. Again... a nice relaxing deep breath... and now begin to focus in on your breathing for a few moments... ignoring everything else around you... all sounds are simply signals to relax... And now let any tension just float away... as you continue to focus on your breathing... your deeper, relaxed breathing... and now just getting centered and continue focusing on your breathing... and simply just allowing relaxation to just happen... effortlessly... magically... automatically...

2. Now, say the following (out loud if you are comfortable): *I feel calm... I feel relaxed... I feel in control... I am calm... I am relaxed... I feel safe... I feel secure... I am confident... I am letting go... as I allow myself to just relax further... and as I let go... all of my muscle groups begin to relax... my jaw relaxes... my whole body is as relaxed as a rag doll or wet washcloth... I feel calm... relaxed... in control... and it feels good to feel good now.*

3. *As all of my muscle groups begin to relax... from head to toe... a wonderful, relaxed feeling comes over me... as I imagine a beam of warm sunlight focuses on my head and spreads relaxation and warmth throughout my entire body... it rids me of all negative thoughts... all negative feelings... and all negative self-talk... leaving me with only positive thoughts and positive feelings... and positive self-talk... I feel calm... I feel relaxed... I am in control... and I persist until I succeed...* Press index finger and thumb together, making a circle, and say again... *I am calm, I am relaxed, I am in control.*

4. *My mind is now relaxed... so completely relaxed and open to receive the helpful and beneficial... and positive suggestions I am about to give myself... for my own highest and best... for my own wellness and success... and happiness.* (Your own personal suggestion goes here, present-tense, positive. Example from Émile Coué: "Every day, in every way, I am getting better and better!")

5. *Taking a deep breath… And exhaling… I feel calm… I feel relaxed… I feel in control… I am calm… I am relaxed… I am in control…* Open your eyes and go about your day! (Emerge self by counting: *One… two… three… four… five*)

Practice! Training your mind requires a small investment of your time each day!

Self-Hypnosis Relaxation Exercise

This is a modified version of the "10 Down to 1 Self-Hypnosis Induction with Muscle Relaxation," originally taught to me by my friend Ron Eslinger, Captain, USN (Retired), and owner of Healthy Visions Hypnosis, in Clinton, Tennessee. It's magical, and with practice, you can apply it anytime you want to go into a light resource state and talk to your wonderful mind. I use this hypnotic induction method with all clients, every week, somewhere in the course of the work we do together. You can use it yourself to help you sleep better! Customize it as you wish. The objective of this is to get yourself into the alpha brainwave state, where you can begin to feed your mind suggestions to help you sleep, or for any other purpose. I suggest you record this into your phone and play it back a few times to get the hang of it. Customize it to suit your needs. Here we go…

Take a deep relaxing breath and now as your body continues to relax more and more… in a moment I am going to count backwards from 10 to 1. As I count you will count with me, but stay one number ahead of me at all times. So, when I say the number 10 you will be thinking of the number 9, and tracing the number 9 over and over, as if tracing it on a marker board. You will stay one number ahead at all times. Every time you inhale, you will think to yourself, *"relax,"* and every time you exhale, you will think to yourself, *"deeper,"* or *"calmer."* So, with every breath you take it will be — *relax*, and *deeper* and *calmer*. Easy, right?

We will now begin. Let's get started.

10– As you breathe deeper now… You are now tracing the number 9 with your eyes, slowly, perhaps using your eyes as the marker, tracing over and over as if writing on a marker board somewhere in your mind. And as you are tracing the numbers, you are thinking, with every breath, "relax," and "deeper." So, you can see, your mind is quite busy at this point. One part of your mind is tracing numbers and another part is keeping track of your respirations. And all the while that you are doing this, your whole body is beginning to relax all over.

9– Relaxing deeper now… now you are tracing the number 8 over and over. You can feel your body relaxing. It's such a nice feeling. Just let all the tensions begin to escape… releasing all stress and tension and anxiety… letting it all go… as you drift to a very peaceful state of relaxation letting a beautiful glowing white healing light glowing down through the crown of your head like a gentle soothing wave of relaxation all the way to your toes cleansing and refreshing. I wonder if you can imagine a hot air balloon carrying away all stress, tension, and anxiety as you give yourself permission to relax deeper as you enjoy watching it drift away, carried away by the wind.

8– Aware of how deep and rhythmic your breathing has become… Now you can feel the relaxation in your neck and shoulders and your neck and shoulders relax deeper and deeper. A nice deep comfortable feeling of relaxation as you continue to breathe easily and comfortably letting all the burdens you usually carry on your shoulders just melt away. Also, any chips you carry on your shoulders can simply be let go… as you imagine yourself unburdened, releasing it all… and relaxing all of your muscles at once.

7– As you slowly trace the number 6 now… breathing to relax… you notice your arms are now relaxing. Everyone relaxes differently and only you know how to relax yourself in this way… Your arms… now they may begin to feel ever so heavy or very light and floaty, whatever you desire, for this is your relaxation. You are always in control, and you will become as relaxed as you let yourself decide to be. Gift yourself this opportunity in this moment right now... let your arms, shoulders, neck, and face just relax.

6– Drawing the number 5 in your mind... you realize the lower these numbers go the more you will let yourself relax, as these numbers go lower and lower, you will feel the relaxation entering your lungs and chest bringing relaxing oxygen into the lungs and transporting to the muscles of the body and cells as you relax deeper and deeper. Imagine for a moment, a cell in your body... every cell in fact... smiling back at you because they are enjoying the increased oxygen you are feeding your body.

5– Now, as you slowly trace the number 4... you can feel it flowing into your abdomen, all of the abdominal muscles are relaxing. You can feel the relaxation going into every organ and nerve within you. You find it so easy to relax yourself any time you choose to... and you could even press your thumb and finger together to anchor this feeling.

4– Now your hips relax, and the relaxation flows down into your legs as they become ever so relaxed. You can feel the relaxation in the thighs as it drifts into the knees and then the ankles and feet. Such a nice peaceful feeling.

3– Now the back is beginning to relax. Starting at your lower back and radiating out to each and every nerve root... slowly relaxing every muscle in your back... Moving again... upward toward your head... to your neck and shoulders all the way into the scalp. Relaxing all of these muscles as you go.

2– Your facial muscles are now relaxing. You can feel it across your forehead, around your eyes and ears, in your cheeks and in the muscles of your jaw, it's such a comfortable feeling to examine and explore. You can even feel your neck muscles relaxing more and more. Bring your attention to the muscles around your eyes... your eyelids... when you are sure your eyelids are completely relaxed... with that relaxation in place... I wonder if you can test them... they will not open... and if they do open... realize you removed the relaxation in order to do so! Relax them down... and just relax deeper.

199

1– Tracing the number zero now over and over very slowly now… feeling relaxed now, feeling good all over in every way. And now, as your whole body begins to take on these very comfortable sensations, relax deeper.

Zzz-Tip: You can add "I am sleeping now" to use this technique for sleep, or you may use any affirmation you'd like in this easy self-hypnosis induction. Enjoy!

When you go to www.iamsleepingnow.com you will receive a link to additional materials to help you sleep better using self-hypnosis as well as for strategies for a happier, healthier, more successful day… and to sleep better and better.

If you need to schedule a personal clinical hypnosis session for sleep, which we offer worldwide, or if you would like to discuss a customized sleep program for your organization, please contact us through the website or call (508) 481-8383.

Printed in Poland
by Amazon Fulfillment
Poland Sp. z o.o., Wrocław
27 September 2023

302af06f-0c90-497a-b2d5-5077cb45f1b2R01